D0514462

Stoma Care in the Community

A clinical resource for practitioners

Edited by
Penny Taylor

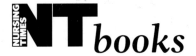

Acknowledgements

Grateful thanks go to Richard and Liz for their patience and support and, when the going got tough, their unfailing encouragement, without which this book may never have reached fruition.

Pictures in Chapter 10 appear courtesy of University Hospital Birmingham NHS Trust and CORCE (Convatec Ostomy Resources Centre Europe).

Every effort has been made to trace copyright holders and to obtain their permission for the use of copyright material. The authors and publishers will gladly receive information enabling them to rectify any error or omission in subsequent editions.

Dedication

This book is dedicated to all the people with stomas whom I have had the privilege to meet and from whom I have learnt so much. Without this sharing of knowledge this book would not be possible

First published 1999 by Nursing Times Books
Emap Healthcare Ltd, part of Emap Business Communications
Greater London House
Hampstead Road
London NW1 7EJ

Text © 1999 Emap Healthcare Ltd.

Printed and bound in Great Britain by Thanet Press Ltd, Margate, Kent.

Cover design by Senate Design Ltd, London.

Typeset by KAI, Nottingham

British Library cataloguing in Publication Data
A catalogue record for this book is available from the British Library.

ISBN: 1 902499 66 2

Contents

Foreword

Penny Taylor

We are now living and working in a changing healthcare climate. In the past the emphasis has been on secondary (hospital) care; times are changing and the shift is towards primary care as the leading force in healthcare provision. Primary Care Groups (PCGs) came into being in April 1999, bringing closer working relationships between general practitioners, nurses and social services to deliver a local service to meet local needs.

People who live with a stoma may spend one or two weeks in hospital but the majority of their time is spent at home cared for as necessary by the new PCG partnerships. Reflecting on this knowledge it seemed the right time to compile a book about caring for people with stomas.

This book has been designed and written as a quick reference guide for nurses in primary care teams to help them care for people with a stoma. This will help the carer make appropriate referrals and improve the quality of care to this group of people.

Stoma care needs to have a multidisciplinary team approach; this book mirrors this belief by having a multidisciplinary writing team. The authors include nurses, an ostomist, a pharmacist, a dietitian, a psychologist, a doctor and a family member of an ostomist. Chapter 1 looks at the history and development of stomas and appliances to set the scene of where stoma care is today. The book can then be divided into two parts: the first part looks at the roles the different specialist nurses play in the care of the person with a stoma, while the second part is devoted to some of the lifestyle issues that occur for this group of people and offers some helping skills. What will become apparent as this book is read is the need for assessment, whatever the situation, as through thorough assessment appropriate and effective care can be offered. This book is intended to be used to aid decision-making when caring for the person with a stoma. It concludes with a list of useful names and addresses.

Throughout this book nursing staff have been referred to as female. This has been done simply for ease of use and readability and does not reflect the fact that nursing staff are made up of both female and male personnel.

Meet the contributors

Barbara Borwell MA(Ed), Dip Coun, Cert. Psychosexual Counselling and Therapy, ENB 216, BCN, FETC, NDN Cert

Starting out as a district nurse, Barbara moved into hospital-based care as a specialist stoma/breast care nurse 19 years ago. She has worked as a lecturer/practitioner and undertaken research on the sexual needs of stoma patients. Much of her work has been published, including a book on developing sexual helping skills, training manuals and an educational game. She has been involved in stoma care courses in Central and Eastern Europe, writes regularly for the nursing press and has given presentations of her work both nationally and internationally. She is currently based at Bournemouth University and is concentrating on her role as nurse consultant and tutor, stoma and breast care.

Susan E. Bridgwater BSc, SRD

Susan obtained an honours degree in Nutrition from Queen Elizabeth College, University of London in 1982 and another in Human Nutrition and Dietetics from the University of North London in 1997. The second degree included state registration as a dietitian. Her first qualified post was at the Kings Mill Centre, Mansfield followed by a full time post with South Birmingham Community NHS Trust. Ostomy patients are often referred to a dietitian for dietary advice and many are very concerned about what they can eat after initial placement of an ostomy. Sound, consistent advice is important to aid recovery and ensure nutritional status is maintained.

Nicholas M. Carter BPharm, MRPharmS

Nicholas qualified as a pharmacist in 1985 and has spent his entire working career in community pharmacy. He has experience in advising a cross section of the public about prescription drugs and the many over the counter drugs available. Many new P.O.M. (prescription only medicines) to P. (pharmacy only drugs) switches in recent years have opened up a new range of more powerful drugs, which can have a variety of side effects.

Catherine M. Cooley *RGN, RSCN, BSc(Hons), MMedSci*

Catherine trained in the West Midlands and initially worked at Birmingham Children's Hospital. During the 1980s she worked as a district nurse in central Birmingham. In 1990 she moved into education, initially as a clinical teacher and then as a Macmillan Lecturer at the Queen Elizabeth College of Nursing. She then became a Macmillan Senior Lecturer in Palliative Care and Oncology at the University of Central England, following the amalgamation of the college into the university. Her areas of interest are cancer pathology and care, malignant and non-malignant palliative care and specialist and advanced nursing practice.

Gail Fitzpatrick *RGN, RSCN, ENB 980, 998, 216, Professional Diploma in Management*

Since 1980 Gail has worked within the paediatric surgical field, with a particular interest in stoma care. She became a clinical nurse specialist in stoma care and bowel management in 1988 and is currently based at the Birmingham Children's Hospital NHS Trust. Her time is divided between the hospital and the community. In collaboration with the University of Central England, Birmingham, she initiated and developed the first paediatric stoma care course in the United Kingdom.

Louise Lewis

Since 1981, Louise has gained considerable experience of stoma appliances working for a number of manufacturers and suppliers. Her roles have included marketing, product development and providing information and advice to patients and healthcare professionals on products and services. She has also been involved in the production of handbooks, directories and leaflets describing surgical procedures and appropriate appliances.

Callum Lyon *MRCP, MA, MB, BChir*

Callum's current post is research fellow in dermatology at the University of Manchester. He is undertaking research into stoma-related skin problems.

Alan Mortiboys

Alan works as tutor for educational development at the University of Central England, Birmingham. He has been a member of the Ileostomy Association for over 20 years and within the association he is active at both local and national level. He is currently developing a programme of accredited training for visitors within ia.

Fran Pinches SRN

After general nurse training at Dudley Road Hospital, Birmingham, Fran qualified as SRN in 1962. From 1963 she worked in the community, first in school nursing and later qualifying as district nursing sister with Staffordshire County Council. She remained in district nursing through the 1970s and early 1980s becoming involved in the mandatory district nurse training as a practical work teacher. In 1985 she changed to the role of clinical nurse specialist, stoma care/coloproctology. Becoming involved in the care of patients, often long term, as district nurse gave her an insight into the family lives of several ethnic groups and an interest in their various cultures and traditions. She has found that by showing an interest and willingness to understand different cultures she has been accepted by even extremely traditional families.

Penny Taylor SRN, SCM, Dip Aroma, Cert Counselling, ENB 216, 998

Penny has worked as a nurse for the NHS for over 30 years, during which time she has seen many changes and reorganisations. She has worked for 13 years as a ward sister on a ward for colorectal surgical patients. In the last 10 years she has set up two stoma care services, the first in a setting of the hospital and the community and the second in a community setting alone. She is currently employed by Southern Birmingham Community Health NHS Trust as clinical nurse specialist, stoma care.

Craig White BSc(Hons), ClinPsyD, AFBPsS, C Psychol

Craig White is Cancer Research Campaign Fellow in Psychosocial Oncology at the Department of Psychological Medicine, University of Glasgow. Dr. White also has honorary clinical appointments with North Glasgow Hospitals University NHS Trust and with Ayrshire and Arran Primary Care NHS Trust. His work regarding psychological adjustment to stoma surgery has been published in surgical, nursing and psychological journals. He is a Fellow of the Royal Society of Medicine and has undertaken higher specialist training in cognitive psychotherapy. His clinical and research interests are in the areas of psychosocial oncology, cognitive therapy, body image and psychological care provision within the NHS. Dr. White is the author of 'Living with a Stoma', a practical guide to psychosocial adjustment following stoma surgery.

1 History and evolution of stomas and appliances

Louise Lewis

A study of history gives us a perspective on the present, and this chapter will take us on a journey from the most primitive responses to trauma and diseases of the bowel to modern innovative surgical techniques. The journey takes us from the most crude of collecting devices, past complex and cumbersome equipment, towards the technical developments which have enabled the production of the more effective and discreet appliances of today. History has seen the emphasis shift from the earliest attempts at curing disease to curing and caring, that is recognising the importance of the patient's quality of life after surgery.

STOMA SURGERY

Stoma surgery prior to the 19th century

Table 1.1 Key developments in stoma surgery prior to the 19th century

55BC–7AD	Celsus	Observations on damage to intestines
1707	Heister	First recorded stoma surgery
1756	Cheselden	Transverse colostomy
1795	Daguesceau	Fashioned colostomy
1799	Larrey	Intestine stitched to abdominal wound

Earliest references to stomas and diseases of the bowel suggest a belief that damage to the small intestine was always fatal, whereas damage to the large intestine could offer a very faint hope of recovery. Celsus (55BC–7AD) wrote: 'sometimes the abdomen is penetrated by a stab of some sort, and it follows that intestines roll out. When this happens we must first examine whether they are uninjured, and then whether their proper colour persists. If the small intestine has been penetrated, no good can be done. The larger intestine can be sutured, not with any certain assurance, but because a doubtful hope is preferable to certain despair; for occasionally it heals up.'

There are occasional references to spontaneous breakdown of gangrenous hernia resulting in stoma formation and references to abdominal wounds that discharged faeces. George Deppe (Fig 1.1) was wounded at the Battle of Ramillies in 1706 and lived for 14 years with a prolapsed colostomy (Cromar, 1968). Despite this limited encouragement there was little surgical development until the early 18th century.

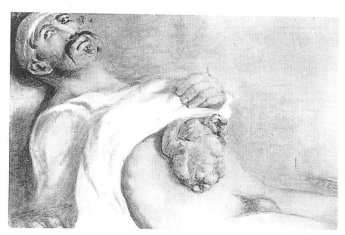

Fig 1.1 George Deppe

A surgeon named William Cheselden described his treatment of a patient, Margaret White (see Fig 1.2). She had an umbilical hernia from the age of 50, and when she was 73 she had a fit of colic and vomiting which caused the hernia to rupture; it prolapsed and became gangrenous. Cheselden had to remove about 26 inches of bowel and formed a transverse colostomy. He wrote that White recovered and lived for many years and that she was taken out of bed and sat up every day (Cheselden, 1756).

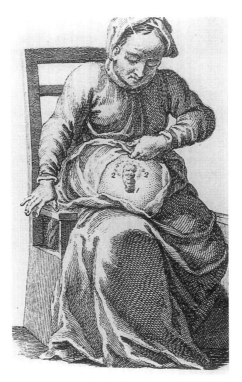

Fig 1.2 Margaret White, the patient of William Cheselden

Two contemporaries of Cheselden, a Frenchman named Henri Le Dran and a German named Lorenz Heister, followed their armies into the battlefield and gained considerable experience of wounds, including those of the bowel. Le Dran had previously observed some patients who, in desperation, attempted to lance what they thought were boils and which were in fact painful inflamed ruptures. According to Le Dran the resulting wound, which was discharging faeces, would sometimes heal if it was cleansed and dressed regularly. He therefore surmised that it was safer to fix injured bowel outside the abdominal wound to stop faeces discharging into the belly and causing peritonitis (Le Dran, 1781).

Heister also described stitching injured gut to the abdominal wall with waxed thread and fixing it firmly with sticking plaster so that the gut could not slip back inside and no faeces could enter the peritoneal cavity. He visited the Dutch camp at Flanders in 1709 and gave a rare description of stoma management: 'there have been instances where the wounded intestine has been so far healed that the faeces which used to be voided per anum have been voided by the wound in the abdomen, which, from the necessity of wearing a tin or silver pipe, or keeping cloths constantly upon the part to receive the excrement, may seem to be very troublesome. But it is surely far better to part with one of the conveniences of life, than to part with life itself.'

As a result of his observations on the battlefields, Heister understood how the facility with which wounded gut adhered to other structures could be used to the patient's advantage (Heister, 1743).

Another instance of both stoma surgery and stoma management was described by a French surgeon called Daguesceau (Cromar, 1968). In 1795 a farmer had pierced his abdomen with a stake after he stumbled while loading wheat onto a cart. Daguesceau created a colostomy from the injury and the man lived until he was 81, managing the stoma by using a small leather drawstring bag as a collecting device.

Dominique Larrey developed his surgical skills on the Napoleonic battlefields and organised a system for dealing with casualties, offering both on-the-spot treatment and evacuation procedures. During the assault on Cairo in 1799 he described the treatment and subsequent recovery of a soldier who had a gunshot wound to the abdomen and intestine. He stitched the damaged intestine to the edge of the abdominal wound which was kept open until the injured intestine healed (Larrey, 1823).

In 18th century civilian life surgeons were slowly becoming more respected. They knew their limitations and, on the whole, were unwilling to take unnecessary risks or use untried techniques, preferring to intervene only to help nature. There were exceptions who were willing to push the boundaries further and suggest more radical intervention. Alexis Littre spoke at the Royal Academy of Sciences in Paris in 1710 and described a post-mortem where he had found the six-day-old baby to have an imperforate anus. He described the rectum as being in two parts joined by threads of tissue; the upper part filled with meconium and the lower part empty. Littre had two suggestions for dealing with this: either open the two closed ends and stitch them together or bring the upper end out on the abdomen to function as an anus (Littre, 1710).

We do not have any records of attempts to try Littre's suggestions until 1783. Antoine Dubois created a colostomy for a three-day-old child who lived for ten days afterwards (Dubois, 1797) and in 1793 a French surgeon called Duret created a successful colostomy on a three-day-old child with imperforate anus – the patient lived until the age of 45 (Duret, 1798).

Stoma surgery during the 19th century

Table 1.2 Key developments in stoma surgery during the 19th century

1815	Freer	First elective stoma surgery
1887	Allingham	Loop colostomy
1895	Paul/Miculicz	Temporary stoma

The first elective surgery recorded in the UK was a colostomy created on a neonate by George Freer in 1815 but the baby died three weeks later (Pring, 1821). These stoma operations in infancy were performed on desperately ill babies with colorectal malformations and, naturally enough at this time, deaths were very common. This type of intervention was slow to gain either professional or social approval.

Professor Gross of Philadelphia, writing in 1859, was astonished 'that anyone possessed of the proper feeling of humanity should seriously advocate a procedure so fraught with danger and followed, if successful, by such disgusting consequences'. He continued: 'I cannot, I must confess, appreciate the benevolence which prompts a surgeon to form an artificial outlet for the discharge of faeces, in a case of imperforate anus.' (Gross, 1866)

Although colostomies were still unusual enough to attract interest on an individual basis, we cannot be sure of the true incidence during Victorian times. Many patients were operated on in their own homes without records being kept. In 1887 William Allingham described his creation of a double lumen loop colostomy held in place with a glass rod. A similar type of temporary diverting procedure is still used today.

A significant step forward in surgery of the large bowel was what became known as a Paul/Miculicz operation, named after two surgeons working in the late 19th and early 20th centuries. It is a temporary stoma in which the diseased colon is resected and the two cut ends are joined together inside the abdomen to make a spur. Later, the continuity of the bowel is restored without further surgery by crushing the spur (Paul, 1900; von Miculicz, 1903).

Stoma surgery in the 20th century

Table 1.3 Key developments in stoma surgery in the 20th century

1913	Brown	Temporary ileostomy
1923	Hartmann	End colostomy
1943	Miller	Proctocolectomy and ileostomy
1950	Bricker	Ileal conduit
1952	Brooke	Eversion ileostomy
1969	Kock	Internal pouch
1978	Parks	Preserved anal sphincter
1980	Mitrofanoff	Internal reservoir for urine

It is not until the early years of the 20th century that moves were made to treat colitis with surgical intervention and ileostomy if medical treatment failed. John Young Brown of St Louis reported in 1913 on the successful management of ulcerative colitis by creating a temporary ileostomy. Continuity of the bowel was restored by anastomosis when he felt the colon had healed. Although this became accepted surgical treatment in the USA, mortality rates were very high as patients were usually desperately ill before referral (Brown, 1913).

The basic technique of colostomy formation has remained unchanged since the middle of the 19th century. We have a description from 1923 of Hartmann's operation for rectosigmoid cancers. This was originally a single operation involving the excision of the upper rectum and sigmoid colon, closing of the rectal stump and formation of a terminal colostomy.

Surgeons were very reluctant to accept ileostomies as permanent and originally it had been intended that ileostomies should be temporary until the disease had been cured and the normal function of the anus could be restored. It became apparent that in many cases not only had the disease returned after rejoining the bowel, but that chronically diseased bowel had a high incidence of malignancy. There seemed no alternative to removing the colon and creating a permanent ileostomy. In the 1930s this was done as a four-stage procedure with several weeks between each stage. First the ileostomy was created, then the right colon was removed, and the proximal end brought to the surface. Then the left colon was removed and the sigmoid was brought to the surface. Finally an abdominoperineal resection was performed. By the 1940s the second and third stages could be done together because of improvements in drugs, anaesthetics and surgical science (Richardson, 1973). In 1943 in Montreal Gavin Miller combined the first two stages of the procedure, performing a proctocolectomy on a young girl with severe ulcerative colitis (Miller, 1949). Miller and his team were the first to perform a one-stage panproctocolectomy, excision of colon, rectum and anal canal and formation of a permanent ileostomy from the terminal ileum.

One of the major drawbacks in creating a permanent ileostomy was the quality of life of the patient after surgery due to inadequate postoperative care. Lester Dragstedt of Chicago used skin grafts around the ileostomy to try to overcome the problem of excoriation but unfortunately these grafts resulted in a high incidence of stenosis, ulceration and sometimes fistula (Dragstedt, 1941). In 1952 Bryan Brooke of Birmingham devised an improved technique for fashioning an ileostomy which involved everting the end of the withdrawn small bowel and suturing it into position to form a 'spout' (Fig 1.3). This helped overcome stenosis and other problems associated with a poorly constructed stoma (Brooke, 1952).

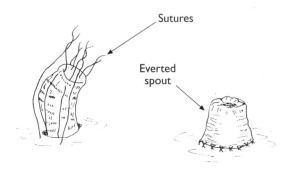

Sutures

Everted spout

Fig 1.3 Eversion of stoma

During the 20th century surgeons became more and more concerned with improving the patient's quality of life after surgery. Some wanted to find alternatives to both the stoma and the necessity of wearing an appliance. New procedures were tried that offered a degree of continence. In 1969 Professor Nils Kock, a Swedish surgeon, reported on his technique of creating an internal pouch from the terminal ileum to act as a reservoir for faeces (Fig 1.4). The pouch is intubated and emptied with a catheter via a nipple valve. This procedure is not suitable for patients with Crohn's disease because of the risk of recurrence within the bowel which makes up the reservoir (Kock, 1969).

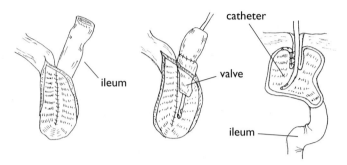

Fig 1.4 'Kocks pouch' – continent ileostomy

In 1978 Sir Alan Parks described his procedure for forming a reservoir from a length of terminal ileum. The ileum is fashioned into a J or W shape, opened and formed into a pouch (Fig 1.5). The tip of the pouch is anastomosed to the anus and, as the sphincters are intact, the patient's continence is restored (Parks, 1980).

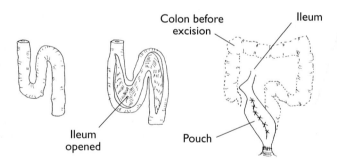

Fig 1.5 Formation of 'Parks pouch'

An alternative to a stoma was sought for those patients who suffered severe faecal incontinence because of loss of the normal function of the anal sphincter. This could be for a variety of reasons such as congenital abnormality, accident, disease or childbirth. A procedure was pioneered in Maastricht and The Royal London Hospital known as dynamic graciloplasty. The gracilis muscle from the thigh is transposed to create a new sphincter, which has to be electrically stimulated to function. This procedure is now available in several centres but patients are warned that it is not always successful.

Urinary diversion

Urinary diversion may be necessary because of cancer and abnormalities of the bladder, to preserve renal function or to restore continence, and there are few records of attempts at intervention before the 20th century. In 1851 John Simon created a channel between the ureters and the rectum to divert a boy's urine but after passing urine in this way for some months he eventually died (Simon, 1855).

In 1911 Robert Coffey diverted the urine by implanting the ureters into the lumen of the sigmoid colon (Coffey, 1911). Technical improvements followed and the wet colostomy or caecostomy came into vogue. The resulting mixture of urine and faeces resulted in frequent skin excoriation and infection and was socially abhorrent.

In 1950 Eugene Bricker from St Louis reported on the improved version of his ileal conduit. Urine passes from the ureters into an isolated section of ileum, one end of which is brought to the surface of the abdomen and a stoma is formed. The continuity of the ileum is restored by anastomosis (Bricker, 1950).

There are three ways of diverting urine: by inserting a tube into part of the urinary tract and changing it at intervals; by diverting the urine internally into another organ, such as the colon; or it may be brought to the surface of the body where it opens by a stoma (Todd, 1978). The ileal conduit remains the preferred type of urinary diversion and different surgeons adopt their own techniques and improvements. Some surgeons implant the ureters separately and others prefer to anastomose the ureters together before implantation.

In the 1980s, in an attempt to avoid the need to wear an appliance, a number of urinary diversions using the Kock ileal pouch were carried out in the USA with some early encouraging results. The Kock Urinary Reservoir is rarely undertaken today because of the technical problems encountered in constructing a continent valve. A French surgeon, Paul Mitrofanoff, has given his name to the Mitrofanoff principle for the formation of a continent pouch, which is the construction of a reservoir, either from the existing bladder or from bowel. The reservoir can then be drained using the appendix to construct a flush stoma which acts as a port for a catheter (Mitrofanoff, 1980). Different surgeons have adapted the technique using alternatives to the appendix such as ureter, vein, urethra, fallopian tube and skin tube.

Stoma surgery has travelled on a long journey since Celsus wrote, 'if the small intestine has been penetrated, no good can be done'. We now know that good can be done and hope for even more in the future. An artificially grown bladder has been implanted in a dog and it has functioned successfully; the next step is an artificially grown bladder implanted into a human (Tomorrow's World, BBC, March 1999).

STOMA APPLIANCES

Stoma appliances prior to the 20th century

Table 1.4 Key developments in stoma appliances prior to the 20th century

1707	Heister	Tins, silver pipes, cloths
1795	Daguesceau	Leather drawstring bag
19th century		Pads, absorbent dressings, binders

Having discussed the tremendous advances in surgical techniques we will now look at something that was essential to the well being and quality of life of the patient, that is the development of an effective appliance. We have brief descriptions of stoma management by the early ostomists. In the 18th century we heard of battle casualties at Flanders who used tins, silver pipes and cloths to collect their faecal output. In the late 18th century Daguesceau gave us his description of the farmer he had operated on who managed by using a small leather bag with a drawstring which he adjusted to fit his stoma.

During the 19th century patients generally relied on pads, absorbent dressings and binders and little had changed at the beginning of this century.

Stoma appliances in the 20th century

Table 1.5 Key developments in stoma appliances in the 20th century

1910	Heavy surgical belts with plastic cups
1930s	Thick heavy rubber bags
1944	Koenig-Rutzen bag
1960s	Thin odourproof disposable plastic bags
	Karaya gum
	Hydrocolloid skin barriers
	Stoma Care Nurses appointed
1980s	Plug system
	Toilet-flushable colostomy bags

From 1910 onwards some patients were managing their stomas by wearing heavy surgical belts with straps and buckles. The belts, which doubled up as support garments, incorporated a plastic cup over the stoma. The patient would line the cup with cotton wool, lint or gauze dressing, which would be changed as necessary. We can only imagine how restrictive and uncomfortable it must have been and how hot and unpleasant in warm weather.

Surgeons faced the dilemma that by creating an ileostomy to cure a patient they would seriously restrict his quality of life afterwards unless they could also offer an effective collecting appliance – one which would cope with the more liquid output of the ileostomist. Therefore they only considered creating an ileostomy if the patient was in a desperate state and this obviously had implications for his recovery afterwards.

In the early 1940s the first rubber bags were manufactured commercially and it became possible to obtain ileostomy appliances. These first rubber bags were a great improvement on what had been available but they still brought major problems for the wearer. They were large and took a considerable amount of time to fit, as they had to be attached to the skin with adhesives. The adhesives used were often so strong that they caused severe irritation to the skin. The bags were used in rotation and carefully washed out, hung up to dry and turned inside out to be powdered. With frequent use the bags began to absorb odours and became smelly.

Some members of the Ileostomy Association, a patient self-help group, wrote about their experiences during this period:

'My ileostomy was born to the days of the non-adhesive bag, when to lie down meant bandages from chest to knees... In the daytime, in order to keep in position a horrible monstrosity of a red rubber smelly bag, one had to wear so stiff a corset that to bend (except at the knees) was impossible. As a single young person, I looked pregnant when returning from hospital.'

'I had my ileostomy given to me in January 1949 by a young surgeon called Bryan Brooke. At that time both ends of the ileum were brought out so I had two stomas. There were no stick-on bags available in this country, but they were being made in America, but to import a set of three into this country cost £15 which was about three weeks' wages then. Many 'do it yourself' efforts were tried out, including cutting up drawsheets and sticking the parts together with Bostik to form bags. Unfortunately when they filled, the joints gave way with disastrous results. Sewing the seams through the Bostik was tried but there were leaks through the stitch holes. Another bright idea was to use a surgical rubber glove with the cuff turned over a rubber ring to form the flange. This was coated with latex and stuck over the active stoma. When the glove filled up it looked like a hand growing out of the stomach, then one of the finger-ends of the glove was cut off and the contents emptied with a milking action. The finger was then sealed with a rubber band.'(Ileostomy Association Midlands Divisions, 1981)

Stoma care for ileostomists took a giant leap forward in 1944 with the introduction of a bag developed in Chicago by an engineering student called Koenig. The Koenig-Rutzen bag was made of thin rubber and was attached to the skin with latex adhesive. The upper opening of the bag had a metal disc covered with rubber and made in different sizes to fit different stomas (Fig 1.6). It brought a new freedom for many patients because it was both discreet and effective compared with what they had before.

Although rubber bags remained popular we were entering the plastic age and people began to see the advantages of lightweight disposable pouches, which did not have to be washed, dried and reused. Attaching both rubber and early plastic pouches to the skin was a complex process, involving the use of strong adhesives such as latex and zinc oxide and belts to apply extra pressure for security (Fig 1.7). Skin allergy and excoriation was common and the fact that these adhesives left behind a stubborn sticky residue added to the problem. Cotton covers in an assortment of colours and patterns were used to make the pouches more acceptable in appearance and also to help prevent excessive perspiration.

There was increasing awareness of the need to protect the skin around the stoma effectively. Karaya gum is collected from trees of the Stericulia Urens family in India and its peculiar property is its enormous swelling power. A teaspoonful, in powder form, placed in a glass of water will form a solid jelly-like mass within a few hours. This property made karaya gum powder useful in the textile, cosmetic and food industry and a very common use was for holding dentures in place.

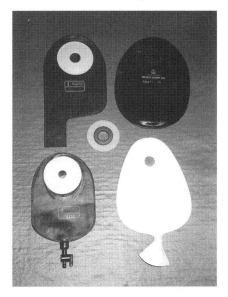

Fig 1.6 Rubber bags

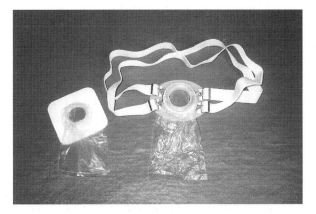

Fig 1.7 Two-piece appliances before Karaya or hydrocolloids

Dr. Rupert Turnbull of the Cleveland Clinic appreciated that its ability to adhere to mucous membranes, such as the inside of the mouth, might prove useful for stoma patients in forming a barrier around the stoma to prevent skin excoriation (Ostomy Quarterly, 1981). Karaya has been used in a variety of forms to protect peristomal skin; it can be sprinkled on in powder form, formed into a separate ring or washer to act as an extra protective barrier, or as an integral part of the appliance itself. For many ostomists karaya brought more effective, longer lasting protection and helped to reduce the amount of skin excoriation.

In the 1960s another giant step forward was taken when the usual polythene pouches were superseded by a thin laminated plastic pouch which was many times more odourproof than its predecessors. Modern stoma appliances are made from several layers of film, each of which imparts different properties to the pouch attempting to ensure that it is odourproof, low noise, soft feel and environmentally friendly. They usually have a layer of soft, water-resistant material on both the front and the back, which makes them more comfortable, reduces noise and improves the appearance of the pouch.

At the same time as the pouches were being improved, more effective skin barriers were introduced which eventually superseded karaya. These barriers were also developed from substances used in dentistry and further reduced the instances of sore skin. We refer to these skin barriers as hydrocolloid adhesives and they are made of carboxymethylcellulose, polyisobutylene, pectin and gelatin – a combination of synthetic and natural materials. They should be strong enough to keep a filled appliance attached to the skin without leaking, even during physical activity and, at the same time, they should protect and maintain the skin area around the stoma. Since the late 1960s manufacturers have continued to research and develop barriers, and modern versions are more flexible, comfortable and durable than their predecessors.

Before the arrival of stoma care nurses in the UK in the late 1960s, patients had looked to surgeons, appliance manufacturers and self-help groups for support, information and advice. Stoma care nurses brought about tremendous improvements in the quality of life of their patients. Among many other things, they encouraged surgeons to improve their techniques and took over the siting of stomas, trying to ensure that the position of the stoma made it as easy as possible for the patient to manage the appliance. At the same time they were taking part in product trials and evaluations and continually pressing manufacturers to make further improvements and additions to the range of products available.

In the 1980s a manufacturer introduced a system described as a plug, which was designed to give the user temporary freedom from wearing a pouch (Fig 1.8). It is suitable for colostomists with a descending colostomy and with regular bowel frequency. When inserted into the stoma, the plug swells like a tampon and can be kept *in situ* for up to twelve hours.

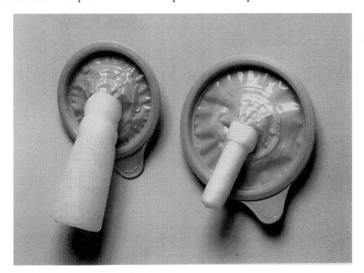

Fig 1.8 'Plug' system – developed in the 1980s and 1990s

Another development during this time was the first colostomy pouch, which was designed to be 'toilet-flushable'. The flushable pouch was welcomed with great enthusiasm by colostomists as it seemed to offer a solution to pouch disposal problems, especially when away from home. Unfortunately a few reports of problems and embarrassment caused by blocked pipes and drains, meant that initial enthusiasm waned and patients were reluctant to risk flushing them away. In the early 1990s a company introduced a more successful product which is a colostomy pouch with a 'toilet disposable' liner. The user removes the liner from the outer pouch and flushes it away in the toilet where it biodegrades in the sewage system.

Modern appliances

Modern appliances are divided into three main groups: drainable, closed and urostomy. Each of these groups of products is available in one-piece and two-piece versions.

- ▶ Drainable pouches are used in the immediate postoperative period and where the faecal output is liquid or semiformed. All ileostomists wear a drainable pouch and some colostomists with a more fluid output need them. They can be emptied via the outlet, which is then sealed with a plastic clip or flexible tie.

- ▶ Closed pouches are worn by colostomists with well-formed faeces and are discarded after use.

- ▶ Urostomy pouches incorporate a non-return valve to prevent reflux of urine onto the stoma, thus reducing the risk of infection. They have a tap for emptying and can be connected to a night drainage system.

One-piece appliances are the most simple to use being lightweight and discreet (Fig 1.9). The pouch incorporates an adhesive flange to secure it to the skin and after use it is removed and replaced by a new one.

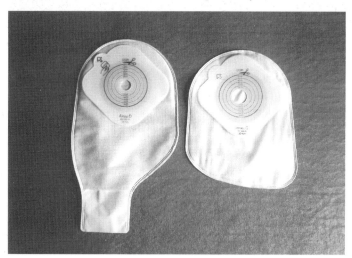

Fig 1.9 One-piece appliances (1990s)

Two-piece appliances (Fig 1.10) have a separate adhesive flange or base plate, which is attached to the skin, and the pouch is then clipped into position on the flange. The pouch is replaced after use but the flange may stay in position for several days. Two-piece appliances reduce the risk of skin excoriation caused by frequent removal of adhesive, and they offer the patient the flexibility of being able to change the capacity of the pouch while keeping the flange *in situ*.

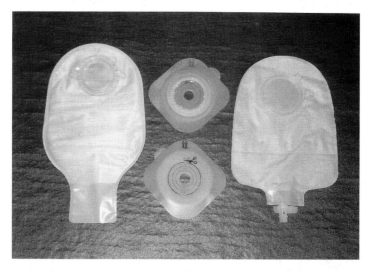

Fig 1.10 Two-piece appliances (1990s)

Pouches are available in both clear and opaque versions. Clear pouches are usually used in the immediate postoperative period or by patients who, perhaps because of poor eyesight, need to feel confident that they have fitted their pouch correctly. Opaque pouches conceal the contents and are more acceptable to the majority of patients.

Patients often experience problems because of flatus, or wind, which can create embarrassment by causing their pouches to 'balloon'. This ballooning can disrupt sleep and can increase the risk of leakage. Closed pouches have long had integral charcoal filters, which allow flatus to be released while absorbing any odour. In the late 1990s modern technology has enabled this solution to be available to ileostomists. Some pouches include a filtration system, which allows the filter to remain effective by protecting it from the more fluid faecal output of the ileostomist.

There is a wide range of accessory products available to patients including pastes, wafers, protective rings, seals and wipes, deodorant sprays, powders and drops, corsets, belts and girdles. These should only be recommended if essential to the patient's stoma care as it is beneficial that the stoma be managed as simply as possible without any unnecessary procedures.

The choice of appliance for a patient is determined by the type of stoma, the faecal output, the site of the stoma, the patient's physical or mental capabilities, the skin condition and sensitivity and last, but by no means least, the patient's choice.

CONCLUSION

This chapter has described the incredible developments in surgery and amazing expansion in the range and quality of appliances available. Tomorrow promises to bring even more improvements and an even better quality of life for those who have a stoma. We owe a great debt to those who have gone before.

REFERENCES

Bricker, E.M. (1950) Bladder substitution after pelvic evisceration. *Surgical Clinics of North America;* 30, 1511–1521.

Brooke, B.N. (1952) The management of an ileostomy including its complications. *Lancet;* ii, 102–104.

Brown, J.Y. (1913) The value of complete physiological rest of the large bowel in the treatment of certain ulcerative and obstructive lesions of this organ with description, operative technique and report of cases. *Surgery, Gynaecology and Obstetrics;* 16, 610–613.

Celsus. De Medicina, English trans. by Spencer, W.G. (1935) London: Heinemann. Cambridge, Mass.: Harvard University Press; 3, 385: Book VII Section 16.

Cheselden, W. (1756) *The anatomy of the human body.* 7th Edition. London: Hitch and Dodsley.

Coffey, R.C. (1911) Physiological implantation of the severed ureter or common bile duct into the intestine. *Journal of American Medical Association;* 56, 397–403.

Cromar, C.D.L. (1968) The evolution of colostomy. *Diseases of the Colon and Rectum;* 11, 256–280; 367–390; 423–446.

Dragstedt, L.R., Dack, G.M., Kirsner, J.B. (1941) Chronic ulcerative colitis. *Annals of Surgery;* 114, 653–662.

Dubois, A. Reported by Allan (1797) *Recueil Périodique de la Société de Médecine de Paris;* 3, 125. (Reprinted in Amussat (1839), p.88.)

Duret, C. (1798) Observations et reflexions sur une imperforation de l'anus. *Recueil Périodique de la Société de Médecine de Paris;* 3, 46. (Reprinted in Amussat (1839) pp. 95–99.)

Gross, S.D. (1866) *A System of Surgery, Vol. 2.* Philadelphia: Blanchard and Lea.

Heister, L. (1743) *A General System of Surgery in Three Parts.* London: Innys, Davis, Clark, Mamby and Whiston. (Original German edition, 1718.)

Ileostomy Association Midlands Divisions, (1981) Newell, A., Pearson, B (eds.) *The first twenty-five years 1956–1981.*

Kock, N.G. (1969) Intra-abdominal reservoir in patients with permanent ileostomy. *Archives of Surgery;* 99, 223–231.

Larrey, D.J. (1823) *Some observations on wounds of the intestines.* Surgical Essays. Baltimore: Maxwell.

Le Dran, (1781) *The Operations in Surgery.* Translated by Gataker, 5th Edition. London: Dodsley and Law. (Original French edition, 1742.)

Littre (1710) Diverses observations anatomiques. *II. Histoire de l'Académie Royale des Sciences. Paris.* 36–37 (Edition published in 1732.)

Miller, G.G., Gardner, C.McG., Ripstein, C.B. (1949) Primary resection of the colon in ulcerative colitis. *Canadian Medical Association Journal;* 60, 584–585.

Mitrofanoff, P. (1980) Cystostomies continente trans-appendiculaire dans le traitement des vessies neurologiques. *Chirurgie Pédiatrique;* 21: 297.

Ostomy Quarterly, Ileostomy Association Midlands Divisions, (1981) Newell, A., Pearson, B (eds.) *The first twenty-five years 1956–1981.*

Parks, AG., Nicholls, R.J., Belleveau, P. (1980) Proctocolectomy with ileal reservoir and anastomosis. *British Journal of Surgery;* 67, 533–538.

Paul and von Miculicz, (1903) Small contributions to surgery of the intestinal tract. *Boston Medical and Surgical Journal* 1903; 148, 608–611.

Pring, D. (1821) History of a case of the successful formation of an artificial anus in an adult, with an account of an analogous operation in two cases by G. Freer of Birmingham. *London Medical and Physical Journal;* 45, 1–15.

Richardson, R.G. (1973) *The Abominable Stoma: A Historical Survey of the Artificial Anus.* Queenborough, Abbot Laboratories.

Simon, J. (1855) Congenital imperfection of the urinary organs treated by operation. *Transactions of the Pathological Society, London;* 6, 256–258.

Todd, I.P. (1978) *Intestinal Stomas.* London: Heinemann.

FURTHER READING

Allison, M. (1998) *An Interactive Guide to Stoma Care Nursing.* CD–ROM, City University, St Bartholomew's School of Nursing and Midwifery.

Black, P.K. (1994) History and evolution of stomas. *British Journal of Nursing;* 3: 1.

Black, P.K. (1999) New developments in stoma appliances and care. *Nurse Prescriber/Community Nurse;* March 1999.

Elcoat, C. (1986) *Stoma Care Nursing.* London: Bailière Tindall.

2 The role of the community stoma care nurse

Penny Taylor

Stoma care is not a new specialist area to nursing – there have been specialist stoma care nurses for over 20 years. This chapter explores the multifaceted role of the stoma care nurse working in a community setting. The aim is to enable the reader to have a better understanding of this specialist nursing post and to acquire the knowledge necessary to use the stoma care nurse to the best advantage of this client group. The sharing of this information may avoid this epitaph:

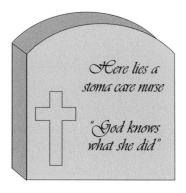

Any stoma care nurse specialist would say their aim was to give a quality service to the people they meet and care for in their professional capacity.

In order to understand how to give this quality service it is important to break down the role into its different components. A widely used model of specialist nursing practice is the one described by Hamric and Spross (1989).

This model will be used for the purpose of describing the functions of the stoma care nurse. What this chapter will not do is debate the issues of specialist practice versus advanced practice; this is well catered for in other books (see Further reading).

Table 2.1 Hamric's Model

1.	Clinician
2.	Consultant
3.	Educator
4.	Researcher
5.	Clinical Leader/Manager

CLINICIAN

The role of the clinician in stoma care nursing is what could be described as the 'master' component. It is the expert knowledge and skills that the stoma care nurse has in the clinical management of people with stomas that enables this specialist nurse to function at a high level of practice. It has been said that specialist posts came into being to improve the quality of nursing care. At all times the stoma care nurse will be acting as a role model to other professionals in the healthcare setting.

The stoma care nurse is in post to provide a quality service to all people with stomas, their families and carers. This service begins at the time a person is told they may need to have a stoma formed. These nurses are in the ideal position to make a thorough assessment of the patient (Wade, 1989). This assessment is the springboard to quality care planning and implementation. The assessment process should begin as soon as possible and should include the following components:

▶ *A full nursing history.* This can be obtained by using one of the nursing models, for example Roper, Tierney and Logan's 'Activities of Daily Living'. Special note will be made about any physical disabilities and how that can impinge on future care of the stoma. The sexuality of the patient needs to be addressed as the formation of a stoma may and can have traumatic effects on sexual function and self-esteem. (These issues are addressed in Chapter 7.)

▶ *A medical history*. This should include past illnesses and also how the present illness presented. At this time a family history could be included.

▶ *Social circumstances*. This enables the practitioner to understand the environment in which the patient lives and at what level they interact with society. If the assessment takes place in the patient's own home there is a greater opportunity to observe this in action.

▶ *Social activities*. The patient will expect to continue to undertake their usual work activities and hobbies. Asking what they do at this time makes it possible to set goals in the postoperative phase of care that are realistic and achievable.

▶ *Psychological assessment*. It is useful at this stage to have an insight into patients' coping strategies. How have they coped with life's stresses? Are there any stressful events happening at present in addition to their illness? This knowledge leads to better care planning and improved patient outcomes. (Psychological care is handled in more depth in Chapter 6.)

In the postoperative phase the stoma care nurse in the community can give detailed information to the patient regarding their disease, stoma formation and type. Discussion on any treatment options can also take place and the implications of this highlighted. These discussions must be a two-way process to enable the patient to make an informed decision about their treatment and care process. Care is planned in conjunction with the patient, their family and any other involved people or agencies. There may be a need for the patient to have several care episodes from the community stoma care nurse in order for this assessment, care planning and decision-making to take place.

Liaison needs to take place between the community stoma care nurse and the stoma care nurse working in the secondary (hospital) care setting. Good communication between primary and secondary care leads to a 'seamless' approach to care.

On discharge from hospital the community stoma care nurse will continue the process of thorough assessment. In addition to the assessment the following areas are observed:

▶ Satisfaction with the stoma appliance.

▶ A scale of physical symptoms is used. It is known that the greater the physical symptoms, the less well the patient is progressing.

▶ Observation of the stoma and wounds are made. The nurse is looking for any problems that may make the stoma management more difficult, for example parastomal hernia or prolapse.

Adaptation to the formation of the stoma will continue for at least one year (Pringle et al, 1998; Wade, 1989.) Therefore regular follow up during this period is recommended. However, stoma related problems may and do occur after this time and the community stoma care nurse is there to help. We are living with an ageing population that is no exception for people with stomas. There may be a time when there is a need for a complex care plan: the stoma care nurse will work with the multidisciplinary care team, aiming to keep the person at home wherever possible.

As part of the ongoing and continuing care of this patient group the community stoma care nurse may facilitate a support group. (The role of self-help and support groups is discussed in Chapter 8.)

The clinical role of the community stoma care nurse is complex. She needs good skills in counselling and communication, expert knowledge in related diseases and stoma care.

CONSULTANT

The stoma care nurse specialist is part of the multidisciplinary team and works in collaboration with each and every one of them. She is a valuable resource, not only to this team caring for the person with a stoma, but the wider healthcare teams and beyond. The stoma care nurse specialist needs to communicate between professionals, and to do this she needs to be credible. This credibility comes through her expert knowledge and skills. Benner (1984) states: 'The expert operates from a deep understanding of the total situation.'

While the stoma care nurse specialist may have a total grasp of the needs in stoma care, others may not, so promotion of the role is vital. Healthcare professionals and the general public need to be aware of the stoma care service – the 'who, what, where, why and when' of it! Without this knowledge the service will not be used to its full potential. Part of this promotion is being available when and where needed, and in a community setting this needs to be flexible. This flexibility needs to be in her attitude to how, when and where service delivery will take place. This often leads to the negotiation of roles with others. She herself may expand her role of practice; some hospital stoma care nurse specialists are pushing forward boundaries of traditional nursing into endoscopy and/or colorectal nurse practitioners. The UKCC's document, 'The Scope of Professional Practice' (UKCC, 1992) states: 'Practice must be sensitive, relevant and responsive to the needs of individual patients and clients and have the capacity to adjust, where and when appropriate, to changing circumstances.' The role of the community stoma care nurse with her consultative hat on lends itself to this statement.

Possessing this expertise puts the specialist nurse in a position to offer peer support and clinical supervision, but in return she herself will need to receive such support. There are various support networks available to stoma care nurse specialists. These may be local, national or international, and there is now the opportunity to become an affiliated member of the Association of Coloproctologists. These kinds of memberships enable the nurse to forge links, increase knowledge and increase dialogue to the benefit of her patient group. This dialogue enables the stoma care nurse specialist to act as a catalyst in problem solving, in particular in complex issues of patient care. Her professional attitude and values enable ideas to be transferred all ways, not only 'top down' but also 'bottom up'. This consultative role is invaluable to patient care, its quality and improved outcomes.

EDUCATOR

Education is a key component of the stoma care nurse specialist's role as a specialist practitioner. Education has traditionally been part of the specialist role and it has important links with the consultative role in the promotion of the service. Through the links forged with other professionals and the already established dialogue they have with other stoma care nurse specialists, education and learning can be easily facilitated. These relationships with others take away many of the obstacles that form barriers for people working in full-time education.

If one were to 'shadow' a stoma care nurse specialist at work it would soon become apparent how much of her time is spent educating. The list of people she engages with for teaching/educating could be endless but for the purpose of this text it could be divided into the following groups:

▶ Patients and families.

▶ Multidisciplinary care team.

▶ General public.

▶ Media.

In order for the stoma care nurse specialist to be an effective teacher she needs to have an understanding of learning. There are three major types of learning:

▶ Affective learning – this is about attitudes and feelings.

▶ Behavioural learning – includes competencies in performing procedures or tasks.

▶ Cognitive learning – includes acquiring information and being able to comprehend it, analyse it and use it in other situations.

The stoma care nurse specialist will also have a comprehension of how learning takes place. This comprehension alone is not enough: she needs to be able to be an effective communicator. Communication needs to be a two-way process between teacher and learner. There also needs to be an understanding of group dynamics in order to formulate a good training session. A good training session will include:

▶ The three types of learning.

▶ Good two-way communication.

▶ An understanding of what each person brings to the session.

As will now be explained, this educator role is not always in the formal setting of a lecture room, but may, for example, take place at a patient's bedside. Much of what we learn is by example and watching others performing, therefore the specialist nurse needs to be a role model. How she undertakes her tasks will reflect the post she is in and her professional integrity is on display constantly. The stoma care nurse specialist needs to frequently self-assess her role and its interaction with others. This enables her to be aware of two things: firstly her own learning needs and secondly how her role is perceived by others. Jarvis and Gibson (1995) state that 'once critical awareness of self-assessment disappears then her professionalism is in danger'.

The clinical nurse specialist has her roots in patient care. This caring role is underpinned by her ability to inform her client group of the skills and knowledge they need to live with a stoma. The educational role with patients and families begins from the time of diagnosis and the necessity for a stoma. It is important for the stoma care nurse specialist to be able to explain the diagnosis, the disease process and the surgery and its implications in terms and language that the lay person understands. This giving, sharing and exchanging of information happens at each contact with the patient. The clinical nurse specialist needs to use her expert skills and knowledge in group dynamics, communication and what blocks learning in order to help the patient have a greater understanding of the situation they face. The diagnosis of ill health, which could be life threatening and/or lead to radical surgery, is a very traumatic time for the patient and his or her family. This in itself will block the communication pathway. Studies by Hayward and Boore (1994) support improved outcomes in recovery: 'Informed talking is more effective than just talking.' This informed talking will continue throughout the visits and consultation that the specialist nurse and the patient have together. Stoma surgery has a great and lasting impact on the patient's lifestyle and possibly that of the family. As time goes on the patient becomes more self-reliant and able to make his or her own decisions. However, there may be a time later in life when a crisis arises and the stoma care nurse specialist needs to be on hand with the information and support required.

'Teaching is of paramount importance if the... nurse is to... improve the care of the stoma patient.' (Elcoat, 1986) This teaching must extend from the specialist nurse to all levels of nursing, from healthcare assistants to student nurses and qualified nurses.

We are living with an ageing population and more people, including those with stomas, are living in sheltered or residential care homes. The majority of workers in these areas are healthcare assistants who may have little or no knowledge of stoma care. This is an ideal opportunity for the stoma care nurse specialist to use her educator role and so improve the quality of care to her patient group. Often healthcare assistants are working towards NVQ Level 2 and 3 and need to gain stoma care knowledge for their portfolios.

Finley (1990) says 'learning the skills involved in stoma care is a cumulative process, occurring over a long period of time and many encounters'. If this is so the stoma care nurse specialist must plan educational sessions throughout the learner nurse training, into the formative years of practice and beyond. Medicine and stoma care are innovative and dynamic and this changing knowledge and skills must be passed on to others.

Nursing does not have the sole right to education from the stoma care nurse specialist: other members of the multidisciplinary caring team need her input. Medical staff can learn stoma care and the patient's needs through constructive discussion with the specialist nurse. There is also interest from medical students requiring information for social medicine projects. Professions allied to medicine may also need input from the stoma care service. It is good practice for the stoma care nurse specialist to capitalise on this thirst for knowledge.

As a stoma care nurse specialist, especially in the community, the aspect of community education must not be neglected. So far education has focused on the patient, the disease and the care requirements, but health promotion must not be forgotten. When a nurse first qualifies for registration one of the competencies she has to undertake is to promote health. The stoma care nurse specialist must actively promote health for her client group and improve the health of the community she serves. For example there are 17,000 deaths per annum in England and Wales (OPCS, 1993) from colorectal cancer. There is much room for improvement in the outcomes of this group of patients. The survival rate for colorectal cancer is poor due to the lateness of the patient presenting to the general practitioner. In turn this is due to the lack of awareness by the general public of the presenting symptoms. Here is an opportunity for the stoma care nurse specialist to make the population more aware of the symptoms and when and where to seek advice. Helpful leaflets are available from the Crocus Trust (see Appendix B).

There is a vast amount of information available through the media and the internet and the stoma care nurse specialist can help the public find a way though this maze. Health promotion in nursing should be proactive not reactive. Now that there is the provision of primary care groups caring for a local population's needs the time is right to encourage the philosophy of promoting a healthier community. Health promotion is about improving the health of a community not just a specific client group.

Education has many dimensions for the stoma care nurse specialist. Some elements of this role take place each day, from role model to teacher in a formal setting to health promoter. Each day will be different but lays the foundation stones of the educator.

RESEARCHER

Research is an important component to nursing today. The stoma care nurse specialist may undertake this role in a variety of ways, however the involvement for each individual practitioner must be reasonable and realistic. In the UK this role is not yet mandatory for the specialist nurse as it is for our American colleagues belonging to the American Nurses' Association. In the future clinical governance and evidence-based practice will be the key to our clinical role. There is a window of opportunity here for the stoma care nurse specialist to influence clinical practice.

Levels of research involvement

Level 1

Practising at this level of competence the stoma care nurse will be able to interpret and evaluate research findings pertinent to the role. She will be able to use her other role of educator as a resource to communicate these finding to others as and when required.

Level 2

The next level of working as a researcher would be to translate these findings into actions and develop innovative practice. This may be taking on board Wade's (1989) findings, for example, and designing an assessment tool for thorough assessment of the stoma patient, or it may be the findings of the Montreux study into the quality of life (Marquis et al, 1995) that is used to map a stoma patient's progress. The stoma care nurse specialist could be involved in conducting research. This could involve helping with recruitment of people into clinical trials of a new stoma product. The manufacturing industry constantly needs to be innovative and dynamic in order to improve the quality of life and care for the stoma patient. This is reliant on a degree of cooperation between patients, stoma care nurse specialists and product manufacturers. Many patients, especially those with colorectal cancer, will be entered into clinical trials for the treatment of their disease. The stoma care nurse specialist's role here is to help the patient understand the need for the trial, the treatment and its implications. It is also important as a specialist nurse to monitor the patient through this period, calling upon the nurse's clinical skills to assess and put in place any necessary interventions, for example nursing needs or referral to another agency.

Level 3

The highest level of research that she could undertake would be to conduct independent nursing research. This involves project design, writing a funding application, getting ethical approval, conducting the study and disseminating the findings. Research by the stoma care nurse specialist can make a substantial contribution to an expanding body of nursing knowledge.

CLINICAL LEADER/MANAGER

Through clinical leadership and management skills the stoma care nurse specialist can influence the delivery of quality patient care. Her resource management skills will give an efficient, cost effective service. Managing the stoma care nursing service may involve human resources: stoma care services could comprise of more than one stoma care nurse and secretarial support. Budget control and financial skills are also an important part of this role. Human resources and stoma pouches are expensive commodities to the health service. However, cost is not the only consideration: stoma pouches must be fit for the purpose they are to be used for and evidence-based practice and best practice must both be considered.

To be a clinical leader the stoma care nurse specialist will facilitate the setting of standards and conduct audit projects for her service. In order for standards to be achievable there needs to be ownership by the staff expected to carry out the care. Staff involvement in the setting of standards will help this process. A tool for this could be a link nurse group, which can be a valuable asset to the stoma care nurse specialist. They provide her with a sounding ground for innovation and can act as a catalyst to change practice, lending support to innovation and change. A specialist nurse has to be a change agent and have an in-depth understanding of change theory. To break the barriers and advance the boundaries of stoma care nursing it is necessary to facilitate change. Communication is of the essence.

 Alongside this skill in communication is the specialist nurse's role as advocate, primarily for her patients. This involves helping patients to make informed decisions and supporting them in communicating that decision to others for whom that decision is relevant. This may include addressing some ethical issues with colleagues from time to time. There could be times when it is necessary to offer clinical supervision to carers when they are involved with complex and difficult emotional cases.

Dilemmas can arise for the stoma care nurse specialist if she manages more than one service. There could be a conflict of interest between the time needed for managing the service and the time needed for clinical practice. Throughout her practice the stoma care nurse specialist needs good time management skills: there is an art to balancing the roles in specialist practice. However, it is through all these roles that she is able to demonstrate her clinical leadership and provide quality nursing care.

Conclusion

As has been explored throughout this chapter the role of the stoma care nurse specialist is made up of a number of roles. These can be broken down into various components, skills and knowledge that add up to a complex and diverse nursing post. Each component has been described individually. They do not stand alone: each is linked with the other. Clinical practice needs research, research needs education and communication skills and, communication skills link back to clinical leadership. The roles that make up specialist practice allow the nurse to develop multiple roles and skills while keeping roots in nursing practice. The basis for community care is quality care: delivering that care at the best point of contact for the patient. It is believed that patients are at their least vulnerable in the own homes and stoma care is therefore less threatening there.

Learning outcomes

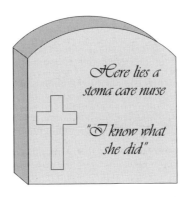

REFERENCES

Benner, P. (1984) *From Novice to Expert*. California: Addison–Wesley.

Cancerlink (1999) *Information for Colon Cancer Awareness*

Elcoat, C. (1986) *Stoma Care Nursing*. London: Bailière Tindall.

Finley, T. (1990) From Text Book to Reality. *Professional Nurse;* Sept. 1990, 617–620.

Hamric, A., Spross, J. (eds.) (1989) *The Clinical Nurse Specialist in Theory and Practice*. 2nd Edition. Philadelphia: Saunders.

Hayward, J., Boore, J. (1994) *Research Classics from the Royal College of Nursing*. London: Scutari Press.

Jarvis, P., Gibson, S. (1985) *The Teacher Practitioner in Nursing, Midwifery and Health Visiting*. London: Chapman & Hall.

Marquis, P., McGrath, C., Marrel, A. et al (1995) International quality of life study in patients with ostomy. *Quality of Life Research Journal;* 4: 5, 459.

OPCS (1993) *Mortality Statistics, Cause, 1993*. Series DM2 No. 32. London: HMSO.

Pringle, W., Swan, E., Wade, B. (1997) *Continuing Care for Stoma Patients*. Presented at the Royal College of Nursing Stoma Forum.

Roper, N., Logan W., Tierney, A. (1980) *The Elements of Nursing*. Edinburgh: Churchill Livingstone.

United Kingdom Central Council for Nursing, Midwifery and Health Visiting (1992) *Code of Professional Conduct*. London: UKCC.

Wade, B. (1989) Ostomates: the case for a thorough patient assessment. *Senior Nurse;* 9: 5.

FURTHER READING

Castledine, G., McGee, P., (eds.) (1998) *Advanced and Specialist Nursing Practice*. Oxford: Blackwell Science.

Humphris, D. (ed.) (1994) *The Clinical Nurse Specialist: Issues in Practice*. Basingstoke: Macmillan.

Myers, C. (ed.) (1996) *Stoma Care Nursing: A Patient Centred Approach*. London: Arnold.

3 The role of the paediatric stoma care nurse

Gail Fitzpatrick

Paediatric stoma patients are a small but significant proportion of the annual national statistics for stoma patients. There are no separate paediatric figures available, but it is estimated that regional paediatric centres see between 40 and 100 new patients each year, excluding gastrostomy and tracheostomy patients. There has been a gradual annual increase in the numbers over the last five years in these regional centres. This may be due to a combination of reasons:

1. Paediatric services have become more centralised in regional centres.

2. An improved survival rate for premature babies and an increased number of premature multiple births, as a consequence of successful fertility treatment, both of which have the potential to increase the incidence of necrotising enterocolitis.

3. The development of continent stomas, antegrade colonic enema and Mitrofanoff procedures – an alternative treatment for faecal and urinary incontinence.

This is reflected in one regional centre's figures for age distribution:

Table 3.1 Age percentage of new paediatric stoma patients

76%	Birth to 2 months
5%	3 months to 1year
8%	2 to 7 years
11%	8 to 16 years

PAEDIATRIC CONDITIONS REQUIRING STOMA SURGERY

Anorectal anomalies

Anorectal anomalies occur in one in 3,000 live births. They can be divided into high and low types, depending on whether the anorectal anomaly is above or below the puborectalis sling. Low anomalies comprise of covered anus, ectopic anus, anal stenosis or anorectal stricture. High anomalies are more complex: the bowel ends as an atresia or continuous fistulas opening (MacMahon, 1991). A fistula presenting in boys is a rectourethral fistula and in girls is a rectovaginal fistula.

Presentation

▶ Absent or covered anus.

▶ Abdominal distension.

▶ Constipation.

▶ Vomiting.

▶ Where there is a fistula, meconium will be passed via the penis in boys and vagina in girls.

▶ Two thirds of these infants will have one or more associated malformations, that is genitourinary, vertebral, alimentary, cardiac, central nervous system. Sacral abnormalities are often associated with neural abnormalities that affect the nerve supply to the bladder and bowel.

Treatment options

Low Anomalies:

▶ Anoplasty.

▶ Anal dilations.

High Anomalies:

▶ Formation of colostomy and mucous fistula.

▶ Pull through procedure using either posterior sagittal approach or abdominoperineal approach. The fistula will also be ligated if present.

▶ Anal dilations.

▶ Closure of colostomy.

Hirschsprung's Disease

Congenital abnormalities occur in one in 5,000 live births (Senyuz et al, 1988). Hirschsprung's Disease is characterised by the absence of ganglion cells in the distal bowel and extending proximately for varying lengths.

Table 3.2 Percentages of affected bowel

60%	Sigmoid and rectum
30%	Rectum only
8%	Whole of colon
2%	Whole colon and small bowel
7%	Familial incidence

Presentation

▶ Delay in passing meconium.

▶ Abdominal distension.

▶ Constipation.

▶ Poor feeders.

▶ Vomiting.

▶ Abnormality most commonly associated with Hirschsprung's Disease is Down's Syndrome.

Diagnosis

Rectal suction biopsies which show ganglia are absent from the submucous and myenteric plexuses and increase in number of nerve fibres in the interface between the circular and longitudinal muscles.

Treatment options

Rectosigmoid Hirschsprung's Disease (short segment)

▶ Rectal washouts followed by one-staged pull through procedure with no colostomy.

▶ Two-staged surgical treatment:

- Defunctioning colostomy.
- Pull through procedure and colostomy closure.

(Pierro et al, 1997)

Total Colonic Hirschsprung's Disease (long segment)

Three-staged surgical treatment:

▶ Defunctioning ileostomy.

▶ Pull through procedure.

▶ Closure of ileostomy.

Modified Duhamel pull through is usually the preferred procedure.

Necrotising enterocolitis

Necrotising enterocolitis (NEC) is the most common abdominal emergency in neonatal intensive care units. NEC is a combination of ischaemia and infective gangrene of the intestine. Its aetiology is unclear but a large proportion of neonates affected have been subjected to some sort of stress, such as prematurity, hyaline membrane disease, umbilical vessel catheterisation exchange transfusion or hypoglycaemia. Mesenteric vasoconstriction in a neonate subjected to stress enables pathogenes to infiltrate the bowel wall and this results in ischaemia and infective gangrene.

Diagnosis

Radiological signs of intramural or intrahepatic gas.

Presentation

▶ Rectal bleeding.

▶ Abdominal distension.

- Bilious vomiting.
- Abdominal erythema.
- Lethargy.

Treatment options

- Rest the intestine, nil by mouth, nasogastric aspiration.
- Broad spectrum antibiotics.

If disease progresses, surgical intervention required. Perforation or peritonitis are possible.

- Laparotomy, ischaemic bowel resected, ileostomy formed.
- Once neonate recovered and thriving, ileostomy reversed.

Meconium ileus

Approximately 10-20% of babies born with cystic fibrosis will initially present with meconium ileus (Mahaffey, 1997). There is a deficiency of pancreatic enzymes released into the intestinal tract which causes the meconium to become thick and inspissated and adheres to the intestinal mucosa resulting in obstruction (Netter, 1979).

Presentation

- Failure or delay in passing meconium.
- Abdominal distension.
- Thick meconium palpable on examination.

Treatment options

- Gastrograffin enema.

If unsuccessful:

- Formation of loop ileostomy to relieve the obstruction and enable stoma washouts to be done.
- Ileostomy reversed once baby is thriving.

Small bowel transplantation

A significant percentage of children with irreversible intestinal failure are dependent on parenteral nutrition. Ten per cent will go on to develop life threatening complications, such as severe problems with establishing venous access, line sepsis and liver disease. Since the 1950s small bowel transplantation has been an alternative treatment for these children. In the early years survival rate was poor until the 1990s when a new immunosuppression drug became available, Tacrolimus (Beath, 1998). It has been essential in allowing small bowel allografts to be tolerated but it also results in a higher rate of infection and lymphoproliferative disease because of the necessary increased exposure to immunosuppression.

Large centres are now achieving three year survival rates of 65% (Langnas et al, 1996). Suitable candidates may be children with short bowel syndrome, intestinal motility disorders or diseases of the intestinal mucosa. (Kocoshis et al, 1997).

Table 3.3

Short gut syndrome	Intestinal motility disorders	Diseases of the intestinal mucosa
1. Congenital small bowel atresias	Hirschsprung's Disease	Microvillous Inclusion Disease
2. Acquired due to extensive bowel resection Volvulus Gastroschisis Necrotising enterocolitis	Pseudo obstruction	Epithelial dysplasia

Depending on the severity of the child's condition they may be assessed for either a combined liver and small bowel transplantation or small bowel transplant alone. After a full assessment of the child's suitability is completed they can go on the active transplant list and await a suitable donor. During the transplant procedure a covering ileostomy is formed to reduce the risks of intestinal leak of the anastomosis and to be able to monitor the condition of the child's donor bowel. The main postoperative complications are related to rejection, infection and nutrition. Some of the many indicators of rejection are increased stomal output and intestinal bleeding, and regular bowel biopsies will be necessary via the stoma to assess the situation (Fitzpatrick, 1996). Depending on the child's progress and state of the large bowel the ileostomy may be reversed six to 12 months after the transplant.

Inflammatory bowel disease

Ulcerative colitis and Crohn's Disease are relatively rare diseases in childhood. Five per cent of Crohn's patients are under the age of five (Fielding, 1986) and 16% of ulcerative colitis patients are under the age of 16 (Dudgeon, 1997).

Presentation

Table 3.4

Ulcerative colitis	Crohn's Disease
20% weight loss	75% weight loss
5% growth failure	40% growth failure
Diarrhoea	Diarrhoea

Treatment options

▸ Conservative medical treatment.

If symptoms are not arrested and the disease increases in severity.

▸ Surgical intervention, formation of ileostomy with partial or total colectomy.

Children with ulcerative colitis may be able to have an ileoanal anastomosis with the creation of a pouch.

Trauma

Puncture or crush injuries to the abdomen as a result of a road traffic accident are the most common form of trauma necessitating emergency stoma surgery. Depending on the injury site the child may have a colostomy, ileostomy or urinary diversion, or a urinary diversion with either of the other two. Wherever possible corrective surgery and stoma closure will be performed.

Rhabdomyosarcoma of the bladder

Rhabdomyosarcomas account for 5-8% of cases of childhood cancer (LaQuaglia, 1997). Rhabdomyosarcoma of the bladder usually occurs in infants and small children.

Presentation

- Bladder outflow obstruction.
- Suprapubic mass.
- Weight loss.
- Malaise.
- Anaemia.

Treatment options:

- Chemotherapy.
- Radiotherapy.
- Radical surgery if the combined chemotherapy and radiotherapy has failed. Surgery involves total cystectomy and formation of bilateral ureterostomies.

Posterior urethral valves

This condition occurs only in boys. It is the result of a developmental abnormality in the region of the verunontanum which leads to the presence of obstructive valvular folds in the urethra (MacMahon, 1991).

Diagnosis

- Routine antenatal foetal ultrasound.
- Postnatal examination reveals large palpable mass due to hydronephrotic kidney and palpable bladder. Associated with posterior urethral valves in vesicoureteric reflux or obstruction at the ureterovesical junction, causing back pressure on the kidneys. Delay in detecting valves is associated with increased damage to the renal tissue.

Treatment options

- Bladder drainage *in utero*.

Or

▶ Insertion of an indwelling catheter followed by fulguration of the urethral valves.

▶ If renal function is grossly impaired, emergency formation of vesicostomy or bilateral ureterostomies. Once valves are fulgurated and renal function is stabilised, stoma can be reversed.

Long term management is necessary as most have associated renal damage and abnormal bladders.

Table 3.5 Top four most common conditions requiring stoma surgery

Anorectal anomalies
Hirschsprung's Disease
Necrotising enterocolitis
Inflammatory bowel disease

TRANSITION FROM HOSPITAL TO COMMUNITY CARE

As far back as 1959 the Platt Report (The Welfare of Children in Hospital) recommended that children should not be admitted to hospital if it could possibly be avoided. Since then several additional reports have been published restating the recommendations and emphasising the need for more community paediatric services to reduce hospital admissions or shorten the length of stay in hospital. It cannot be argued that stoma patients require essential periods of hospitalisation but early discharge can be possible with the help of community nursing services. In Britain the mean length of stay for 0–4 year-old children steadily declined from seven days in 1974 to four days in 1989–90 (Department of Health, 1991). Early discharge from hospital has many advantages for both the child and the family, but it does mean that while the child is in hospital everything happens at a fairly rapid pace and the parents go through a steep learning curve. Usually the parents are quick to learn and adapt to caring for their child's stoma and are always eager to go home. Despite feeling fairly confident on discharge, once home the parents often feel anxious, isolated and unsure of their ability to care for their child's stoma. The first couple of days following discharge are a crucial time when parents need adequate support and reassurance.

PROVISION OF COMMUNITY CARE

The number of paediatric stoma care nurses in Britain is relatively small and they are usually based at regional paediatric centres. A recent research study (Rogers, 1997) looked into who cared for the stoma children in the community where there was no paediatric stoma care nurse:

Table 3.6 Percentage of referrals

50%	Local adult stoma nurse
25%	Paediatric community nurse
25%	District nurse or combination of all three

Often children's conditions are complex resulting in a large number of additional personnel being involved in the child's care (Fig 3.1).

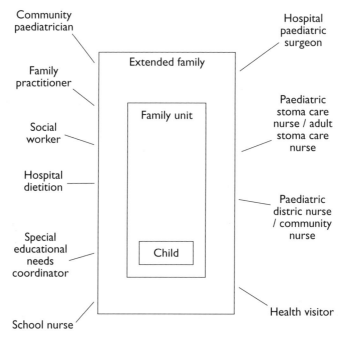

Fig 3.1 Example of potential personnel involved in child's care

There will always be advantages and disadvantages for having so many people involved in one child's care.

Table 3.7

Advantages	Disadvantages
1. Wealth of available knowledge and expertise. 2. 24 hour cover.	1. Conflicting advice 2. Confusion or overlap of job role and responsibilities 3. Parents overloaded with people. Home can feel like an extension of the hospital.

To ensure that the team enhances patient care in preference to hindering it, a 'named' person should be appointed to coordinate the child's care and ensure good communication channels within the team.

COMMUNITY CARE

For parents to feel confident about caring for their child's stoma and to cope with any stoma-related problems, such as peristomal soreness, granulation tissue or stoma prolapse they require ongoing practical support, information and reassurance. In addition to the practical management of the stoma the parents often have other associated concerns and ask similar questions.

Can my child go in the bath?

Yes, with or without the bag on. Reassurance may be needed to confirm that water will not seep into the body via the stoma once the bag is off. Baby oil in the water should be avoided as it will prevent the bag from sticking. Ordinary baby bath is ideal.

The bag keeps blowing up with wind

Paediatric bags do not come with integral filters, but there are individual filters to stick on, which can be just as effective for deflating a child's bag.

Can my baby be immunised?

If the baby was premature or anoxic at birth it is best to consult the baby's paediatrician first. Otherwise the baby can be immunised at the usual times.

How do I explain to siblings about my child's stoma?

Honest and simple explanations are often the best approach. In addition play can be used to enhance the explanations as that is an extremely effective way for a child to learn. There are many storybooks, colouring books and stoma dolls available that can be used.

Why does my child need sodium supplements?

Babies with a stoma, particularly an ileostomy, can lose additional sodium from the body. This can be monitored by measuring the urinary electrolytes. Without adequate levels of sodium the baby will not thrive, so if the levels are low oral sodium supplements are given to replace the lost sodium.

Why does my baby need special lactose free milk?

Babies who undergo small intestinal resection and formation of a stoma may develop a lactose intolerance. This is due to mucosal damage occurring at the time of surgery and lactase is the most susceptible enzyme to such an insult (Jones et al, 1985) resulting in the malabsorption of lactose from the infant's feeds. It is usually a temporary problem and once the stoma is closed and the baby has recovered normal formula milk can be tried.

Should my child wear a bag over a vesicostomy?

It does not matter either way. If the child is still in nappies it may be easier to just protect the peristomal skin with protective wipes or barrier creams and wear double nappies at night to prevent any wet beds. In older children or where a younger child is consistently getting wet clothing it is best to wear a bag over the vesicostomy. Often it is best to let the child dictate whether they wish to wear a bag or not. Vesicostomies are usually formed in the toddler age range as a very temporary stoma.

Can I get financial help?

If the child has had a disability for longer than three months and requires a substantial amount of additional care in comparison to another child of the same age, they will be entitled to Disability Living Allowance. Claims can be made through local Disability Living Allowance offices. Payments are made weekly and claims are reviewed annually. There are also various other organisations, such as the Family Fund, which might be able to help.

Can my child go to nursery and school?

Yes, the child's health visitor will often be able to advise of a local nursery school that will take children with special needs. Before the child is due to transfer from nursery to school it is advisable to approach the headteacher of the school selected to discuss their needs. Most schools are helpful and the transfer should take place without major problems, provided careful liaison has been maintained. If after discussion with the school obstacles are raised or school admission is refused, parents should be reminded that there is no good reason why a child with a stoma or incontinence should not go to a mainstream school. Under the 1981 Education Act there is a requirement that, whenever reasonably practicable, children with special educational needs should be educated in mainstream schools alongside other children. This means that the Local Education Authority (LEA) has the obligation to ensure that the child's needs are met as far as possible in the mainstream school. If the child's needs are still not met parents have the right to request that the LEA undertakes a multidisciplinary assessment of the child. It is a legal requirement that parents be involved in this. The 'assessment' consists of interviews and visits. At the end of the procedure the LEA issues a statement setting out the conclusions and, if there are special needs, what it intends to do to enable these needs to be met. The statement is maintained by the LEA and is transferable from one area to another if the child moves house. The statement procedure may take months and it is advisable to start this process well in advance of the time when the child is due to start school.

ANAL DILATIONS

Children with anorectal anomalies usually require anal dilations following corrective surgery (Paidas and Pena, 1997). The medical staff will perform the first dilation approximately seven to 10 days after the operation. Thereafter parents can be taught to perform the dilations.

Aim: To dilate a narrow or newly created anus to enable the child to pass faeces without discomfort.

Psychological preparation and support

Parents find the dilations the most difficult task they have to perform throughout their child's treatment (Forest-Lalande, undated), often commenting that caring for the stoma is easy in comparison to the dilations. They may express shock at the size of the dilators, dislike the appearance of the healing anus, get upset if the child cries or be very frightened of hurting their little one. Fathers may also raise concerns that someone outside the family unit could misinterpret the situation and accuse them of child abuse. The parents need to be aware of the importance of the dilations and if not correctly done or not done regularly may compromise the success of the surgery. The dilations can be taught in the child's home as long as the parents are given ongoing guidance, support and reassurance. A small percentage of parents feel unable to perform the dilations and must not be pressurised to do so. Alternative arrangements can be made for a community nurse to visit daily to perform the dilations (Fig 3.2).

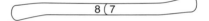

Fig 3.2 Hagar Dilator

Medical instructions required

▶ Dilator size.

▶ Frequency of dilations.

▶ Distance dilator to be inserted (dependent on child's anatomy, i.e. site of stricture or anastomosis).

Equipment

▶ Correct size, Hagar dilators.

▶ Lubricating jelly.

Procedure

▶ Position infant on back, remove nappy, clean bottom.

▶ Lubricate the first inch of the Hagar dilator with lubricating jelly.

▶ Lift the infant's legs upward, flexing the knees towards the abdomen.

▶ Gently insert the Hagar dilator, rotate clockwise 90°.

▶ Slowly withdraw dilator.

▶ Wipe away any surplus lubricating jelly from the anus.

▶ Reposition and comfort the infant.

▶ Wash dilator in soapy water, store in a safe, dry place.

Table 3.8 Potential problems

Problem	Cause	Recommendation
1. Rectal bleeding	Trauma due to dilations.	If bleeding does not stop spontaneously seek medical advice.
2. Difficult to dilate	Fibrous ring or stricture.	Use dilator one to two sizes smaller then try correct size again. If it remains difficult inform medical staff.

Table 3.9 The four main areas of community care

1. Psychological support
2. Practical skills and help
3. Educational input
4. Financial support

BOWEL MANAGEMENT

It is not uncommon for a proportion of children with congenital anorectal anomalies or Hirschsprung's Disease to suffer from faecal incontinence several years after the stoma is closed. The problem of faecal incontinence is a devastating one both for the child and the family. These children benefit from individualised bowel management programmes. These programmes can be initiated and supervised by specialist paediatric nurses working in the community.

After thorough assessment a bowel management programme is agreed which is acceptable to the child and family.

There are three main options:

1. Laxatives.

2. Colonic cone irrigation.

3. Antegrade colonic enema.

Laxatives

Aim: For the child to produce a regular bowel motion preventing faecal retention and subsequent soiling due to 'overflow' diarrhoea.

Each child needs a different amount and type of laxative. The amount required can only be determined by trial and error. The child and family are counselled and educated to follow a specific laxative and toilet training regime. Constant reassessment and fine adjustments of the programme are essential in achieving faecal continence.

Colonic cone irrigation

The colonic cone irrigation technique is a useful alternative method for achieving faecal continence in a small percentage of children who have failed to achieve continence using laxatives, suppositories or enemas (Shandling and Gilmore, 1987). Children born with anorectal anomalies, Hirschsprung's Disease, spina bifida or idiopathic constipation can be suitable candidates.

Contra indications are the presence of a megacolon, gut motility problems, inflammatory bowel disease, or anal stenosis.

Aim: To empty the rectum and prevent soiling (Paidas and Pena, 1997).

Psychological preparation and support

Colonic cone irrigation can be viewed as intrusive and potentially distressing to both child and parents, but must be weighed against the psychological effects of a child who constantly soils. With careful handling, sensitivity and continued support the colonic cone irrigation can revolutionise a child's life, giving them new found confidence and improved self-esteem. It is essential that the child fully understands the procedure, its benefits and agrees for it to be carried out. Consent must be obtained from both the child and parent. It is beneficial to teach the child and parents the procedure in the community as the child will be more relaxed and feel safer in their own surroundings (Fig 3.3).

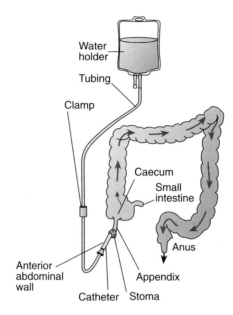

Fig 3.3 The cone irrigation set

Equipment

▶ Cone irrigation set.

▶ Lubricating jelly.

▶ Measuring jug.

▶ Kitchen salt (not low sodium salt).

▶ Lukewarm tap water.

▶ Bathroom hook.

Procedure

▶ Prepare irrigation fluid by mixing lukewarm tap water and kitchen salt in the measuring jug. Fluid volumes vary depending on the child's weight – 20ml water for every kilogram of body weight, plus one teaspoon of salt for every 300ml of water.

▶ Pour fluid into the water holder and release clamp to allow fluid to run through. Expel the air and re-clamp.

▶ Suspend water holder on bathroom hook about one metre above the child's hip level. This allows fluid to run smoothly with minimum pressure.

▶ Lubricate tip of cone with lubricating jelly.

▶ Position child, lying on his or her left side with both legs flexed. This places the descending colon at the lowest point.

▶ Insert tip of cone into anus.

▶ Release clamp and allow fluid to run in slowly. This usually takes two to three minutes. If leakage occurs gently insert cone further in until leakage stops.

▶ Once all the fluid has run in re-clamp tubing and remove cone.

▶ Quickly sit child on the toilet, preventing any unnecessary accidents.

▶ The child will need to sit on the toilet for at least 30–45 minutes to evacuate their bowels and ensure that all the fluid is expelled.

▶ On the toilet the child's abdomen can be gently massaged to assist the evacuation.

▶ Wash cone irrigation set with warm soapy water. Rinse thoroughly and hang up to dry.

▶ The colonic cone irrigation needs to be repeated on a regular basis. The frequency of the procedure will vary from child to child. To prevent soiling the procedure may be required daily, on alternate days or every third day.

Table 3.10 Potential problems

Problem	Cause	Recommendation
1. Rectal bleeding	Trauma due to cone insertion	Stop cone irrigation for a week. If bleeding persists, seek medical advice.
2. Poor results, soiling	Faecal retention	Give oral laxatives until clear.
3. Retention of irrigation fluid	Incorrect fluid concentration	Check water and salt quantities and re-adjust.

Problem	Cause	Recommendation
4. Poor compliance	Boredom	Organise for child to play games, do puzzles or read while sitting on the toilet.
	Embarrassment or dislike	Discuss with medical staff child's suitability for an 'ACE' procedure.

Antegrade colonic enema

The antegrade colonic enema (ACE) provides an alternative system for a few children who remain incontinent despite trying various bowel management programmes or children who have been successful with the cone irrigation but now want a less invasive system.

Suitable candidates may be children with anorectal anomalies, Hirschsprung's Disease, spina bifida or chronic idopathic constipation. Contraindications are the presence of gut motility problems and mega rectum. The technique was first developed by Mr P Malone in 1990. One end of the appendix is re-implanted in a non-refluxing manner into the caecum and the other end is brought out onto the abdominal wall as a continence stoma.

Aim: To provide a catheterisable channel through which antegrade washouts can be given to produce colonic emptying and prevent soiling (Malone et al, 1990).

Due to the child's underlying condition they usually have already undergone some form of abdominal surgery. In the past it was thought to be sensible to perform an incidental appendectomy at this time due to the risks of developing appendicitis, whereas the argument today is against this practice because of the potential of the appendix valve being used in surgical reconstruction (Wheeler and Malone, 1991). If the child has already had an appendectomy paediatric surgeons are able to utilise a piece of bowel to create a catheterisable channel or a caecostomy button may be inserted into the caecum (Fig 3.4).

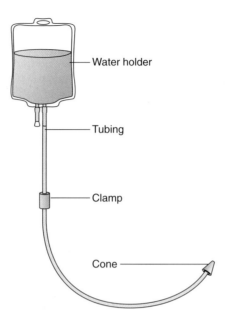

Fig 3.4 Antegrade colonic enema

Psychological preparation and support

Before any decision can be made the child and parents must be given every opportunity to explore all the options, have a full understanding of the ACE procedure and what it entails, in particular the ongoing time commitment. It is often beneficial for the child and parents to meet another child who has already got an ACE. After surgery a catheter is left in the ACE stoma for anything between two and six weeks to allow the channel to heal. During this time it is not necessary for the child to stay in hospital. Once the catheter is removed the child can be taught to pass the self-lubricating catheter. The ACE irrigations can start from the fifth day after the operation using the indwelling catheter, eventually progressing to the self-lubricating catheter.

Equipment

▶ Phosphate enema.

▶ Measuring jug.

- Kitchen salt.
- Teaspoon.
- Lukewarm water.
- Irrigation set (similar to the cone irrigation set, replacing cone for a catheter tip connector).
- Self-lubricating catheter (size 8–10).
- Bathroom hook.

Procedure

- Prepare irrigation fluids, two solutions required.

  Solution 1 – Phosphate enema diluted with equal volume of salt solution.

  Age seven or younger, 30ml phosphate enema.

  Age seven to 10, 50ml phosphate enema.

  Solution 2 – Salt solution 10ml per kilogram of body weight. Salt solution 300ml lukewarm tap water mixed with 1 teaspoon of kitchen salt.

- Pour Solution 1 into the water holder, release clamp to expel air and re-clamp.
- Suspend water holder on bathroom hook about one metre above child's hip level.
- Prepare self-lubricating catheter.
- Sit child on toilet.
- Insert catheter into ACE stoma, connect end to irrigation set.
- Run Solution 1 in followed directly by Solution 2 and re-clamp.
- Remove catheter and irrigation set. Throw catheter away.
- Wash irrigation set with warm soapy water, rinse thoroughly and hang up to dry.

Additional information

For the first month the antegrade colonic enema needs to be performed daily, then on alternate days or every third day if no soiling occurs. After a couple of weeks it may be possible to combine Solution 1 and 2, as long as no soiling occurs. To prevent the occurrence of stoma stenosis, a catheter is passed into the stoma twice a day. After a couple of months it can be reduced to once a day.

Table 3.11 Potential problems

Problem	Cause	Recommendation
Difficulty in passing catheter	Stoma stenosis	Increase frequency of stoma dilations. If no improvement, may need stoma refashioning.
Retention of irrigation fluids	Incorrect fluid concentration	Check fluid concentrations and adjust.
Poor results, soiling.	Faecal retention	Adjust fluid concentrations or change type of solutions used, i.e. 'Klean Prep' or give oral laxatives.
Leakage from stoma	Faecal fluid refluxing	Refashion stoma.
Sore perianal skin	Localised infection	Swab site. Give course of oral antibiotics if infected.
Nausea or pain during irrigation	Bowel spasm or phosphate toxicity	Stop irrigation for a few minutes until pain subsides. Restart slowly. If no improvement, reduce volume of phosphate enema used.
Poor compliance	Boredom	Organise for play activities for child while sitting on the toilet.

Table 3.12 The three stages of bowel management

1. Holistic assessment
2. Agree bowel management programme
   a. Laxatives
   b. Colonic cone irrigation
   c. Antegrade colonic enema
3. Ongoing monitoring programme, adjustments and support

CONCLUSION

Having an ill child can be traumatic and stressful at the best of times but for parents with a child requiring repeated hospitalisation and surgery the experience can be much more difficult to cope with. The support received from staff can make all the difference (Stewart, 1990).

REFERENCES

Beath, S. (1998) *The Birmingham View On Small Bowel Transplantation In Children.* Birmingham Children's Hospital.

Dudgeon, D.L. (1997) Ulcerative Colitis. In: *Surgery of Infants.* Philadelphia: Lippincott–Raven.

Department of Health (1991) *Health and Personal Social Services Statistics for England.* London: Government Statistical Service.

Fielding, J.F. (1986) The relative risk of inflammatory bowel disease amongst parents and siblings of Crohn's Disease patients. *Journal of Clinical Gastroenterology;* 8, 60.

Fitzpatrick, S.G. (1996) The child with a stoma. In: *Stoma Care Nursing: A Patient Centred Approach.* London: Arnold.

Forest–Lalande, L. (undated) Ostomy care in paediatrics: Particularities. WCET; 106.

Kocoshis, S.A., Reyes, J., Todo, S. et al (1997) Small intestinal transplantation for irreversible intestinal failure in children. *Digestive Diseases and Sciences;* 42: 10, 1997–2008.

Langnas, A.A.N., Shaw, B.W., Antonson, D.L. et al (1996) Preliminary experience with intestinal transplantation in infants and children. *Paediatrics;* 99, 443–448.

LaQuaglia, M.P. (1997) Rhabdomyosarcoma and non rhabdomyosarcomatous sarcomas. In: *Surgery of Infants and Children.* Philadelphia: Lippincott–Raven.

MacMahon, R.A. (1991) Urinary tract infection and abnormalities of the urinary system. In: *An Aid To Paediatric Surgery.* 2nd Edition. Churchill Livingstone.

Mahaffey, S.M. (1997) Meconium Syndrome and Cystic Fibrosis. In: *Surgery of Infants and Children.* Philadelphia: Lippincott–Raven.

Malone, P.S., Ransley, P.G., Kiely, E.M. (1990) Preliminary report: The Antegrade Continence Enema. *The Lancet;* 17: 336, 1217–1218.

Ministry of Health, Central Health Services Council (1959) *The Welfare of Children in Hospital (The Platt Report).* London: Ministry of Health.

Netter, F.M. (1979) Diseases of the lower digestion tract. *The CIBA Collection of Medical Illustrations.* Vol. 1 Digestive System. New York: CIBA.

Pierro, A., Fasali, L., Kiely, E. et al (1997) Staged pull through for recto sigmoid Hirschsprung's Disease is not safer than primary pull through. *Paediatric Surgery;* 32: 3, 505–507.

Poudas, C.N., Pena, A. (1997) Rectum and anus. In: *Surgery of Infants and Children.* Philadelphia: Lippincott–Raven.

Rogers, J. (1997) Who cares for children with stomas? *Eurostoma;* 23, 12–13.

Senyuz, O.F., Danismend, N., Erdogan et al (1988) Total intestinal aganglionosis with involvement of the stomach. *Paediatric Surgery;* 1988: 3, 74.

Shandling, B., Gilmore, R.G. (1987) The enema continent catheter in spina bifida successful bowel management. *Paediatric Surgery;* 22: 3, 271–273.

Stewart, A.J. (1990) Mums and dads need care too: supporting parents of babies in neonatal units. *Professional Nurse;* 5, 660–665.

4 The role of the community nurse

**Tracey Allen, Vanessa Foxall, Christine Thompson,
Maureen Appadu, Jill Doyle, David Harries,
Frances Roberts**

> 'Nursing is primarily assisting the individual, sick or well, in the
> performance of those activities contributing to health, or its recovery
> (or to a peaceful death) that he would perform unaided if he had the
> necessary strength, will or knowledge. It is likewise the unique
> contribution of nursing to help the individual be independent of such
> assistance as soon as possible.'

(Henderson, 1960)

In this chapter we will discuss the role of the district nurse in caring for
stoma patients in the community and consider how this role relates to the
specialist stoma nurse and other nurses and healthcare professionals
working in primary care. The chapter includes an overview of district
nursing and presents a nursing assessment through the framework of a
nursing model.

We acknowledge that there are many nurses working in a community
setting who also care for stoma patients before and after surgery and that
district nursing intervention will not be needed for every individual.
Practice nurses provide a useful source of help and advice for ostomists on
a wide range of issues. They may also refer patients on to other healthcare
professionals for help in particular areas. Younger children and
adolescents may be referred to the paediatric nursing service and/or the
school nursing service, as appropriate. In some cases care may be shared
between community nurses from different disciplines.

AN OVERVIEW OF DISTRICT NURSING

District nursing comprises a complex and subtle blend of activities which is centred on the patient and family, and which embraces the wider community and other health and social care providers. McDonald et al (1991) pointed out that reductions in acute hospital services and the movement from secondary to primary care bring issues of role definition as well as changing caseloads to district nursing teams. Skill mix and staffing levels have also come under scrutiny influencing role and grade distributions within teams (NHS Executive, 1992).

The caseload of the district nurse is generally defined as being derived from the population for which she has designated responsibility (ENB, 1991). This is usually the GP practice population. A recent survey of 24 community trusts indicated that nearly all of the district nursing services were GP attached or aiming to become GP based in the near future (McDonald et al, 1997).

The gold standard of district nursing care is to facilitate and promote optimum independence and well-being of the patient. Ross (1991) identified that rehabilitation and the promotion of health and self-care are two of the key functions of district nursing.

Community nurses to a greater or lesser extent become part of the patient's social and support network. The community nurse will recognise that in some cases people will want to take a full and active part in their own self-care or participate fully in the care of others. However, some people find themselves completely unprepared. Similarly nurses need to respect the lifestyle choices and health beliefs of the patient and their family.

Each person's capability to deal with the practical aspects of a stoma will vary but, whatever the level of intervention, the knowledge that the nurse has, and the willingness and ability to provide intimate care for the stoma, will go some way towards eventual acceptance and rehabilitation. Clinical skills are also essential to the teaching that will facilitate that rehabilitation. The nurse's skill in practical procedures and her knowledge of the normal appearance and action of a stoma lends her the credibility to advise within the client's own home and to recognise and anticipate potential problems that may affect recovery.

Nursing assessment

On legal, ethical and professional grounds nurses need to carefully consider and reflect upon the care they plan, implement and evaluate. In attempting to explain and define the nursing role and contribution to the care of a patient with a stoma, practitioners can turn to nursing theory to provide a way forward and use the framework of a nursing model.

Nursing models are attempts to explain the theoretical values that are held to be fundamental to the practice of nursing. These values add to the uniqueness and richness of a profession that is committed to developing its knowledge base from practice (Pearson et al, 1992). Important concepts within nursing models are those that concern the person receiving care, the environment in which care is given, how health or nursing needs are defined and the nature or purpose of nursing. It has been suggested in the literature that nursing itself has a therapeutic effect borne out of the nurse's personality and knowledge (Travelbee, 1968).

There is no universal agreement on the single best model for community nursing. Some practitioners may favour one particular model over the rest, whereas other community nurses may reflect elements of several models to inform their practice. Evidence of adapting aspects of a model in the design of nursing assessment and care plan documents is commonplace within district nursing but it should not be assumed that their underlying theories have been universally embedded in real life practice.

 Common examples of care advocated by a particular model include activities of daily living (Roper et al, 1980) or the universal self-care requisites of Orem (1991) which readily lend themselves to a structured assessment framework.

In Orem's model nurses should attempt to identify the personality and characteristics of patients and relatives that may affect the nursing situation. These may include passivity, anger or grief and will need to be sensitively explored. Unresolved emotions may affect partnership and collaboration within the nurse-patient relationship. The community nurse will need to use her interpersonal and observational skills to elicit this information (Kavanagh, 1991).

A case history together with an example of a nursing assessment and care plan have been used to explain the many elements of caring for a patient who has recently been discharged from hospital following formation of a stoma. The assessment framework is based on the model developed by

Virginia Henderson (1960) whose definition of nursing is quoted at the start of this chapter. This model was chosen because Henderson emphasises the nursing role in maintaining independence or restoring an individual's independence in meeting fundamental needs (Aggleton and Chalmers, 1986).

Table 4.1 Description of model

Care is organised around four important nursing concepts:
1. The person being nursed
2. The environment in which care is given
3. The health status of the individual
4. The nature of nursing

Henderson describes 14 fundamental needs, which are common to all individuals, sick or well. An assessment of Mrs. Jones' care needs using Henderson's model as a framework is produced on page 64.

The fundamental needs identified by Henderson are in priority order and relate closely to the work of Maslow (1970). Maslow recognises that physiological and safety needs should be met first since only then can a person concentrate his or her resources on meeting their psychological and social needs. This approach seemed particularly appropriate in respect of the following case history.

CASE HISTORY

Mrs Jones is an 80-year-old widow who has no children and lives alone in a small terraced house. Her only relative is a nephew who lives 40 miles away. As a result of reduced mobility and limited income she has gradually become more isolated at home.

Mrs. Jones' first contact with the district nursing service followed a request for help with faecal incontinence. On assessment it was found that she had a three-month history of a constant desire to open her bowels and frequent passage of small liquid motion. She had become incontinent of faeces and subsequently was sore and uncomfortable. On examination by the GP she was found to have a large mass in the rectum.

A diagnosis of carcinoma of the rectum was made following referral to a consultant. Mrs Jones underwent radiotherapy and an abdominoperineal resection of the rectum and formation of colostomy was performed. Post operatively Mrs Jones was slow to recover and demonstrated reluctance in becoming involved in the care and management of her stoma. She was eventually discharged from hospital seven weeks after her operation and referred to the care of her GP and the district nursing team.

Table 4.2 Assessment of nursing needs

Fundamental need	Normal	Present
Breathing	No breathing difficulties usually. Mrs Jones is a non-smoker.	No problems identified.
Eating and drinking	Previously healthy appetite, eating three meals a day and snacks. Likes fresh fruit and vegetables. Drinks about six cups of tea each day and juice for breakfast.	Appetite reduced, not enjoying food. Afraid of the effects of fruit and vegetables on stoma. Has lost weight. Doesn't feel up to preparing food.
Elimination	Problems began six months ago with bowels, which lead to operation and stoma. Before that bowels were 'normal'. No urinary problems.	Reluctant to manage stoma. Finds it complicated and there is too much to remember. Worried she can't get supplies. Doesn't like changing bag downstairs and concerned about disposal of bags.

Fundamental need	Normal	Present
Mobilisation	Was starting to experience difficulty with stairs due to arthritis. Tending to use furniture to support herself getting round the house. Hasn't been out alone for past year. Friend takes her shopping.	Unable to get upstairs. Has chemical toilet downstairs in front room, which is now a bedroom. Using a Zimmer frame to aid walking. Has difficulty rising from chair.
Sleep/rest	Normal pattern is to sleep well and undisturbed throughout night.	Sleeping in front room and finds sleeping difficult due to worry about future. Waking three to four times in night.
Dressing/clothing	Likes to get dressed each day and has no difficulty managing clothing.	Managing to dress each day and adjust clothing for stoma. Wears suitable unrestricting clothes.
Temperature	No central heating but gas fires in each room. Manages to keep warm	Managing to adjust heating and keep warm. Expressing worries about paying heating bills.
Washing hair/skin	Enjoys a daily bath and a visit to the hairdresser each week. Friend takes her in the car.	Feels dirty, conscious of odour from stoma. Experiencing difficulty getting upstairs to use bathroom.
Safety/environment	Able to negotiate moving around house using furniture sometimes. Taking stairs slowly.	Loose mats and rugs on floor increasing risk of falls. Feels vulnerable at times but wants to stay at home.

Fundamental need	Normal	Present
Communication	Mrs Jones' main relationship is with her close friend. Has no problem with hearing or sight. Has never had a telephone but likes to write letters.	Feels increasingly isolated since returning from hospital. Says she has lost confidence. Reluctant to discuss stoma or illness.
Worship	Attended local church services every week with her friend and likes to be involved in church activities including lunch club.	Feels that she can't do this any more because of the stoma and how other people may react.
Work/occupation	Always been a housewife and takes pleasure in keeping a neat home, preparing meals etc.	Hasn't been out of house since returning from hospital. Feels cut off.
Play/recreation.	Daily outings or trips with friend. Involved in lunch club and church activities.	Doesn't want to go out in case stoma acts or smells.
Learning/discovery	Used to enjoy going out and seeing friends, watching TV, listening to radio and reading papers and magazines.	Feels as though she has lost interest in former activities.

Table 4.3 Plan of care

Fundamental need	Goal	Nursing intervention
Breathing	No problems identified	
Eating and drinking	Restore nutritional status Reverse weight loss	Advice/education re. balanced diet and use of nutritional supplements. Refer to home care for help with cooking/ shopping or 'meals on wheels'.
	Reduce anxiety over which foods to eat	Evaluate/advise on the effect of certain foods on stoma activity.
Elimination	Acceptable conditions for changing stoma	Establish routine times for changing stoma to avoid visitors. Reassurance re. smell and use of deodorising spray.
	Confident in managing stoma independently	Use teaching plan in easy stages to acquire skills with back up information. Establish process for obtaining supplies. Maintain communication with stoma therapist.
	Allay fears of stoma bag disposal	Arrange clinical waste disposal.
Mobilisation	Improved mobility will include getting upstairs, walking around the house and getting up from the chair	Review management of arthritis through liaison with GP. Refer to OT for assessment of mobility. Refer to social services for assessment for stair lift or downstairs bathroom conversion.

Fundamental need	Goal	Nursing intervention
Sleep/rest	Improved sleep pattern through reduction of anxiety	Review of sleep problems with GP.
		Give time to express anxiety, reassure and support.
		Refer to social services re. personal alarm system.
Dressing/clothing	No problems identified	
Temperature	Optimal financial support in place	Arrange financial assessment via social services.
Washing hair/skin	Improved perception of body image	See intervention for mobilisation.
		Give education/ counselling re. body image.
		Assessments for assistance with personal hygiene – home care, private resources or short–term intervention from nursing auxiliary.
Safety/environment	Risk of falls reduced	Advise on removing loose mats.
		Reinforce use of walking frame.
		Arrange OT assessment of home environment.

Fundamental need	Goal	Nursing intervention
Communication	Improved confidence in self-image	Provide encouragement to rejoin activities.
Worship		
Work/occupation		Ensure stoma appliance is well fitting and use of filter to diminish smell.
Play/recreation		
		Reassurance and counselling support from nurses and stoma therapist
Learning/discovery	Regain interest in usual life activities	Liaise with GP and stoma therapist concerning future outlook.
	Improved outlook on the future	Provide reassurance and emotional support.
		Refer for psychological support if needed.

PLANNING CARE

The presence of a stoma changes the way in which the individual manages the process of defecation and can permanently change the individual's perception of their body image. This can affect all areas of a person's usual physical, social and emotional functioning and affect their day to day activities, interactions and relationships. There may be a resulting loss of personal privacy and independence, which can have a profound impact on the individual's sense of dignity and self-esteem. These issues have been addressed specifically within the plan of care but will now be considered more broadly in terms of implications to district nursing.

Personal and emotional care

The nurse's attitude and approach will convey powerful information to the patient who may be watching for signs of distaste or reluctance in handling bags or cleansing the skin around the stoma, or simply being in close physical proximity to the patient.

The patient may have fears for the future, which may be related to their diagnosis and also to their ability to cope when the nurses are not around. They may fear the reactions of family and partners and wonder if life will ever be normal again. The nurse should be willing to explore these areas with the patient and allow time for the patient to express their feelings.

Promoting recovery and rehabilitation

The district nurse can provide a wide range of equipment for the home to assist the recovery and independence of the patient. This may include aids to daily living and mobility equipment. When assessing which items of equipment to provide careful thought needs to be given as to where the equipment or aids are to be used and to client acceptability. A chemical toilet or commode, for example, may meet a short term need for patients who need toilet facilities close to hand but this may prove undesirable to the client as indicated in the assessment example. In the longer term it may be appropriate to consider adaptations that will enable a patient to gain access to their usual bathroom facilities, such as a stair lift or the fitting of a downstairs bathroom and toilet.

Stoma appliances and supplies

The specific needs of the stoma patient will include providing information on how to obtain supplies of stoma bags and appliances. The patient may also need advice on appropriate disposal. In some circumstances this may include referral to the local environmental health agency for provision of clinical waste services.

Education and teaching

The community nurse cannot promote the goal of patient advocacy and choice without the ability to teach. It is only by learning the skills necessary to deal with a stoma, and by accumulating the related knowledge, that the individual will be able to take control of their lives again, and maximise their independence and normality.

At times of stress the ability to retain information can be reduced. The district nurse needs to be able to recognise barriers to understanding and learning, and be prepared to invest time, patience and understanding to overcome these obstacles. Interpersonal skills are vital in this area and the degree of trust the professional engenders in the client will have a large impact on the eventual outcome. It is within this sphere that the district nurse can also deliver appropriate health education.

Liaison

Within the community care setting the nurse is a member of the primary healthcare team as well as being part of a wider network of multidisciplinary/multi-agency care.

Community nurses need the professional and personal skills to work effectively with other health professionals and social care providers. It is particularly important that the nurse and the patient's GP share information concerning the patient's needs and progress. In this way the patient can feel confident in being cared for by people who communicate with each other and will not receive conflicting information and advice. It also allows the patient to have a clear understanding of the available support services and other providers involved in their care. This is important if they are to feel in control of their situation and be able to participate fully in decision-making and in exercising choice.

Referral to another discipline

Community nurses require a clear understanding of their role and that of others. Where identified problems fall outside the scope of nursing or when the input of another health or social care professional is identified, the community nurse will need to make the appropriate referral.

The nurse must also be aware of her own limitations in skills and knowledge in that area of stoma care and be prepared to involve health care professionals with specialist knowledge. Many trusts employ a stoma nurse specialist who provides a valuable service by advising and supporting nurses, doctors, patients and families both in hospital and in the community, thus improving the quality of care for patients.

Reassessment and discharge

The individual's progress along the road to rehabilitation and recovery must be reviewed at regular intervals and the care plan modified appropriately. The client–nurse relationship is paramount in this process, as is the understanding that any reduction in nursing visits following reassessment does not represent a withdrawal of the service but is the result of a successful transfer of ability from nurse to patient.

It is important for the client to have ongoing access to professional advice and support after the district nursing intervention has ended. In the event of a change in condition, or a problem with daily management, the individual should have a named contact person to call on. Some ostomists may wish to become a member of an ostomist support group and the nurse will be able to advise them on this.

It is important that both client and nurse view discharge as a desirable and eventual goal from the outset, and representative of a successful outcome. An episode of community nursing care involves the building of close relationships on both sides, which can sometimes complicate the quest towards maximum independence. The nurse should have nurtured the client's confidence in their ability to cope with their stoma, and in their knowledge that healthcare professionals are still there if they are needed.

PROFESSIONAL EDUCATION AND DEVELOPMENT

The requirement of nurses to maintain their knowledge and skills and to deliver a safe standard of care is made explicit in the professional codes of practice (UKCC, 1992).

It would be inappropriate, if not impossible, for the specialist stoma nurse to directly manage the care of all stoma patients. However, the opportunity for community nurses to care for patients with a stoma may not arise on a regular basis. This presents a challenge to nurses in terms of maintaining confidence and competence in their role and in keeping up to date with current treatment recommendations in this area of practice. Training days, courses, seminars, conferences and professional literature are all important in terms of helping practitioners to acquire, develop and expand their knowledge base.

The UKCC (1995) has stated that clinical supervision will play an increasingly important part in ensuring safe and effective standards of care. It would seem that clinical supervision is integral to the process of increasing professional self-regulation, which has been highlighted by the present government's plans for managing quality in the NHS (Department of Health, 1998).

Community practice teachers

Within the clinical area the community practice teacher has a significant and influential role in supporting and developing practice. Community practice teachers (CPTs) are district nurses who have a broad understanding of clinical practice within their speciality and an in-depth knowledge of the local population and related health, social and economic issues. Jarvis and Gibson (1985) identify that CPTs embrace a dual role of practitioner and teacher operating at the interface of theory and practice and that the role is a specialist occupation in its own right.

The community practice teacher can act as a role model and teacher in the care of patients with a stoma in the community setting to nursing students and other members of the nursing team. Community practice teachers are expected to have the skills and knowledge to link theory to practice and to facilitate an effective learning environment where professional development needs can be met alongside the delivery of patient care.

The role of the link nurse

Many trusts use link nurse meetings as a forum for the exchange of information between the specialist nurse and nursing teams both in the community and in the hospital setting. In this way the specialist nurse acts as a consultant in the management of care, is available to discuss problems and difficulties, and can disseminate education to inform practice.

A link nurse for each team or area is identified to meet regularly with the specialist nurse and other link nurses and becomes a resource for her team by cascading information from the link nurse meetings.

Belbin (1993) suggests that a well-balanced team is made up of a reasonable number of participants with a diversity of talents and team roles. Diversity within the team, if directed effectively, creates opportunities that can greatly increase the team's potential. The link nurse is then a member of both her immediate nursing team and the link nursing team and needs to be able to contribute effectively to both.

As a member of the immediate nursing team the link nurse acts as a resource for her colleagues concerning the care of patients with a stoma and related issues. She may also share relevant information within the wider primary care team and the newly forming primary care groups. As a link nurse team member she can contribute ideas and suggestions that may improve the finding, sharing and disseminating of information concerning stoma care and patient management. For example, link nurse meetings can be held to review educational materials, to produce clinical guidelines or to set up a system for clinical supervision of practice to support the development of competence and confidence in practice.

The role of the specialist nurse within the link nurse team is important. The success of the link nurse model in developing and disseminating knowledge for practice in our experience is strongly influenced by the approach, strengths and skills of this individual.

The nurse specialist acts as an advocate to link nurses and patients aiming to achieve the most appropriate management strategy for their needs whilst ensuring an effective use of her expertise (Storr, 1998). It has been suggested that in order for theory to advance, the clinical nurse specialist is dependent upon questions arising from link nurses which current research has not covered, thus emphasising the reciprocal relationship between theory and practice (Charalambous, 1995). Link nurses can also be influential in encouraging colleagues to adopt more effective ways of working as change agents within their practice area.

In addition to sharing and disseminating information, link nurses may become involved in developing educational courses and in teaching locally or more formally. The role may also include auditing and collection of data.

Gibson (1989) has identified motivation and enthusiasm as essential requirements of the link nurse role. Although Gibson was writing about continence promotion and management, the same principles hold true for stoma care. Gibson warned that travelling distances and unpredictable workloads may prevent the regular attendance of community nurses at meetings.

A review of the link nurse role suggests that involvement offers the individual opportunities for personal and professional learning and development and the opportunity to shape and develop practice. It is important to recognise that there must also be a wider commitment to disseminating and sharing knowledge and information with colleagues and members of the primary care team if the changing needs in stoma care nursing are to be met.

RESPONSES TO CHANGE IN THE COMMUNITY

The cycle of change within the NHS continues to affect nurses working in the community as well as nurses in the acute, private and independent sectors. Specialist nurses are also influenced by these changes as they often work across primary and secondary care settings and traditional professional boundaries.

Concerns about the cost of care, fragmentation of care delivery and variations in care standards across the country have lead to successive government reviews of the NHS. The present government has replaced the internal market created by the NHS and Community Care Act (1990b) with 'integrated care'. Integrated care is 'based on partnership and driven by performance', according to the strategy set out in the White Paper, 'The New NHS: Modern, Dependable' (1998). Some of the most important changes arising from the new NHS strategy are the development of primary care groups and the emphasis on quality driven by the National Institute for Clinical Effectiveness and the introduction of Clinical Governance (Department of Health, 1998).

The government has made it clear that it wishes to encourage an NHS based on partnership, where staff can work effectively and efficiently in teams within and across organisational boundaries. This has lead to the call for integrated nursing teams that can share expertise and pool knowledge and skills. However, it has been noted that practice and community nurses may regard each other as threatening (Wood, 1994).

Conflict is divisive and creates the potential for clinical errors, which can lead to adverse care outcomes for patients and a poor healthcare experience. Integrated care is seen to rely on models of education and training that enable staff to gain a clear understanding of how their roles fit with other health and social care professions and providers.

The government has also signalled its support of recent developments where nurses have led practice by setting up nurse managed clinics and district wide specialist services. This indicates clear approval and encouragement for nurses to develop defined roles based on their professional expertise and knowledge. From this basis there is the potential to support research and development in patient care, lead developments in care and service management, strengthen nurse education and contribute to frameworks for professional self regulation.

CONCLUSION

The role of district nurses in the appropriateness and effectiveness of district nursing intervention is an important consideration for primary health care management in today's NHS. District nurses clearly have a role in promoting the recovery and rehabilitation of patients following lifestyle changes resulting from illness or injury.

The aim of this chapter has been to demonstrate that the scope of district nursing is wider than the perceptions of a procedure-focused 'hospital care' at home service. The care of a patient with a stoma is one example of an area of community nursing practice that can demonstrate the depth and breadth of the district nursing role to its full extent.

REFERENCES

Aggleton, P., Chalmers, H. (1986). *Nursing Models and the Nursing Process.* Basingstoke: MacMillan Education Ltd.

Belbin, M. (1993) *Team Roles at Work.* Oxford: Butterworth Heinemann.

Charalambous, L. (1995) Development of the link nurse role in clinical settings. *Nursing Times;* 91, 11.

Department of Health (1990b) *NHS and Community Care Act.* London: HMSO.

Department of Health (1997) *The New NHS: Modern, Dependable.* London: HMSO.

Department of Health (1998a) *A First Class Service. Quality in the New NHS.* London: HMSO.

English National Board (1991) *Criteria and guidelines for taught practice placements for district nursing students.* Circular 1991/05/MB. London: ENB.

Gibson, E. (1989) Co–ordinating continence care. *Nursing Times;* 13, 4.

Henderson, V. (1960) *Basic principles of nursing care.* International Council of Nurses: Geneva.

Jarvis, P., Gibson, S. (1985) *The Teacher Practitioner in Nursing, Midwifery and Health Visiting.* London: Chapman Hall.

Kavanagh, S.J. (1991) *Orem's Model in Action.* London: Macmillan Education.

Maslow, A. (1970) *Motivation and Personality.* 2nd Edition. London: Harper Row.

McDonald, L.D., Addington–Hall, J.M., Hennessy, D.A. et al (1991) Effects of reduction of acute hospital services on district nursing services: implications for quality assurance. *International Journal of Nursing Studies;* 28, 247–255.

McDonald, A., Langford, I., Boldero, N. (1997) The future of community nursing in the United Kingdom: district nursing, health visiting and school nursing. *Journal of Advanced Nursing;* 26: 2, 257–265.

National Health Service (NHS) Executive (1992) *The Nursing Skill Mix in the District Nursing Service.* Value for Money Unit Study. HMSO: London.

Orem, D.E. (1991) *Nursing: Concepts of Practice.* 4th Edition. New York: McGraw–Hill.

Pearson, A., Punton, S., Durant, I. (1992) *Nursing Beds: An Evaluation of the Effects of Therapeutic Nursing.* Harrow: Scutari Press.

Roper, N., Logan, W.W., Tierney, A.J. (1985) *The Elements of Nursing.* 2nd Edition. London: Churchill Livingstone.

Ross, F. (1987) In: Littlewood, J. (ed.) *Recent Advances in District Nursing.* Longman Group UK Ltd. Churchill Livingstone.

Storr, G. (1988) The clinical nurse specialist: from the outside looking in. *Journal of Advanced Nursing;* 13, 265–272.

Travelbee, J. (1968) *Review of Interpersonal Aspects of Nursing.* New York: Pitmans.

United Kingdom Central Council for Nursing Midwifery and Health Visiting (1992b) *The Code of Professional Conduct.* 3rd Edition. London: UKCC.

United Kingdom Central Council for Nursing Midwifery and Health Visiting (1995) *Clinical Supervision for Nursing and Health Visiting;* Registrar's letter 24 January.

Wood, N., Farrow, S., Elliott, B. (1994) A review of primary health–care organisation. *Journal of Clinical Nursing;* Vol. 3.

5 Palliative care

Catherine M. Cooley

The aim of this chapter is to enable the nurse to identify the important issues surrounding care and management in the delivery of palliative care to the patient with a stoma.

Palliative care is the care given to those patients for whom cure is no longer a possibility (World Health Organisation, 1990). The most important consideration for these individuals is that the life span that is left should be of the highest quality. When considering treatment and care the benefits must always outweigh the disadvantages and nurses play a pivotal role in acting as the patient's advocate. They need to ensure that what the patient feels is to their advantage is not subsumed by the need of the professional to do their best for the patient. Palliative care is a rapidly developing field of practice where its image as being the soothing hand and 'tender loving care' has changed. It has become a field of practice in which some of the treatments previously utilised to cure are being modified to palliate (Dunlop and Kaye, 1997).

Stoma patients that the community nurse is likely to care for in the palliative care phase of life fall into two categories. First, those who had their stoma formed previously to treat acute 'benign' disease, such as: ulcerative colitis or Crohn's Disease, and who have now been diagnosed with a life limiting disease. Second, those who have had a stoma formed to 'palliate' symptoms, for example in obstruction. The commonest pathology associated with a life limiting diagnosis and a stoma is the patient diagnosed with colorectal cancer.

Throughout this book many issues are highlighted which are extremely important for effective palliative care delivery, such as psychological support, sexuality, pharmacology and pain management. In this chapter we consider the issues for the community nurse caring for the palliative care patient in their home setting, identifying the importance of teamwork in palliative care and considering some of the symptom control issues. We also look at some of the other 'treatment' modalities that may be utilised to manage symptoms, such as chemotherapy and radiotherapy.

KEY ISSUES IN PALLIATIVE CARE

Although palliative care has been practised since ancient times, its development as a specific discipline began only 30 years ago (Twycross, 1995). The resulting benefits for patients have been in enhancing relief from difficult distressing symptoms and improving their quality of life. The introduction of palliative medicine as a distinct discipline in 1989 and the increasing numbers of nurses, occupational therapists, physiotherapists and social workers educated and specialising in this field have enabled the development of a multiprofessional approach to care management (Waller and Caroline, 1996). These improvements in care management have been best demonstrated in the care of people with advanced cancer.

It is said that most patients would prefer to die at home (Doyle, 1996). The fact remains, however, that while patients may spend 90% of the last year of life at home, fewer people than ever actually die there (Doyle, 1996). The reasons for this are complex and varied, the most common being poor symptom management, especially pain, lack of planned care, slow response to emergencies and the quality of communication and co-operation between the many healthcare professionals. However, it is also worth identifying that family distress and fear of being alone with the dying patient are also key reasons for hospital admission even when the best care package is in place.

Some patients with cancer may have access to their local hospice, which can advise on symptom control, and spiritual and psychological care. Many of these hospices have a home care team who will work closely with the community team enabling the patient to remain in their home setting. There has recently been a further development with the advent of 'Hospice at Home' services in which a team from the hospice delivers continuous care to the patient within their home, rather than moving them into a hospice. These are still fairly rare but have the potential to support patients who wish to die at home.

A TEAM APPROACH TO PALLIATIVE CARE

The improved effectiveness of treatments has led to a situation in which the palliative care phase of the patient's life has increased. While it is acknowledged that patients will probably still die from their disease, the length of survival and the potential quality of survival have become difficult to determine. For the community nurse the importance of information regarding the prognosis and potential problems which could occur is paramount (Randles, 1998).

Feeling confident enough to offer advice but being aware of limitations is a key issue in the delivery of palliative care (Jenkins, 1997). It is important for the patient and their relatives/carers to feel confident in the abilities of their professional carer and truth and trust are important in the development of a therapeutic relationship. Acknowledging a lack of knowledge, while being able to identify other team members who have specialised skills, improves this relationship.

It can be argued that through their training community nurses are well placed to offer information and emotional support to this patient group (Grande et al, 1996). However, patients can also get additional support through access to specialist nursing care from the stoma care nurse specialist and the palliative care nurse.

Those patients who have had a 'palliative' formation of a stoma will normally have been recently referred to the specialist stoma care nurse. For patients who have had their stoma for a considerable length of time there may already be a well-established relationship. However, if the patient has been coping well with the stoma for many years and has lost contact with the specialist stoma care nurse, it is important for the community nurse to establish the specialist nurse involvement. The specialist stoma care nurse will often have direct access to the surgeon who performed the surgery leading to the formation of a stoma. The information from the surgeon may influence the subsequent care and management of the patient.

The palliative care nursing team may include a Macmillan nurse, Marie Curie nurses and hospice nurses who have all developed their knowledge and skill in the specific field of palliative care. The palliative nurse specialist will be able to advise on general management of difficult symptoms and will be able to collaborate in accessing resources for the patient with cancer. The palliative nurse specialist may also be aware of the information regarding prognosis, support networks and resources that have been offered to the patient.

All nurses also have a pivotal role in the psychological care of the palliative patient and in supporting the families. Most patients' needs are met by the development of an open relationship in which the nurse is able to offer the time to listen to fears and concerns. However, it is clear that some patients have deeper psychological problems that may need the support of a trained counsellor, psychologist or a specialist nurse with experience of these situations.

Relatives often approach the practice nurse to seek advice and to discuss anxieties. A close working relationship between the team will ensure she is fully informed of the patient's situation and can build on the advice being offered by the team attending to the patient's day to day needs.

The palliative care patient will come into contact with vast numbers of individuals who will offer their advice and support; this can sometimes become overwhelming and confusing for the patient (Table 5.1). It is often necessary for the community nurse to protect the patient from well meaning but excessive help.

Table 5.1 The 'Caring' Team

Stoma Care Nurse	Community Nurse	Palliative Care Nurse
GP	Surgeon	Ward Nurse
Social Worker	Hospice Team	Chaplain
Occupational Therapist	Physiotherapist	Oncologist
Palliative Care Consultant	Friends	Health Care Assistant
Radiographer	Radiotherapist	Health Visitor
Practice nurse	Family	Neighbours

What is clearly identified is the need for a good communication network to be established, especially between the patient, family and healthcare professional and between the professionals (Ingham and Coyle, 1997). This will ensure that whoever is delivering the care, in whatever setting, is fully aware of the patient's medication, 'treatment' discussions, prognosis and wishes.

One of the identified ways of improved communication is a good understanding of the roles of the other individuals involved. Another way, which is gaining favour in the field of cancer care, is the development of patient held records. These expand the community nursing home records to records which cross the boundaries between settings and professionals.

Patients who do not have a cancer diagnosis but are in need of palliative care may not have the same degree of access to the palliative team, despite that fact that their needs may be almost identical. The GP, practice nurse, community nurse and specialist stoma care nurse become the key professional carers and are able to utilise their palliative care skills across the pathologies.

Symptom identification and management

Symptom assessment and management are an important part of palliative care. Effective pain management is one of the key requirements, as pain is one of the most feared symptoms for the dying individual (Twycross, 1997). For the palliative care patient a range of 'treatments' and complementary therapies can be utilised. Listening to the patient, identifying their wishes and utilising their own knowledge of 'self' will enable better care management to be developed.

As the patient's condition deteriorates bowels can become troublesome and irregular, odour may become more apparent and appliances may need to be reviewed (Randles, 1998). Anorexia, fatigue and nausea may all add to the symptoms experienced by the patient.

The causes of symptoms are either the disease progression, the psychological state of the patient or the drugs utilised to relieve other symptoms. One of the most difficult drug related problems is how to minimise the link between good pain control and the potential side effects of opioids, especially constipation. For the palliative care patient, with or without a stoma, the symptoms and psychological distress caused by constipation can be overwhelming. Pro-active prevention is important; those patients who have had their stoma for some time will be aware of what has an effect on normal function and will be able to identify at an early stage if they are becoming constipated. Those patients for whom the stoma has been the choice for palliation of obstruction will not have had the time to become experienced in early identification of potential problems. Constant and careful monitoring of output will alert the community nurse to possible problems and ensure they are dealt with before they become an acute problem.

Ensuring that patients are always prescribed a laxative when taking mild or strong opioids should now be common practice; ensuring these laxatives are increased as the pain relief is increased and assessment that the laxatives are still appropriate is not always so well undertaken. Pro-active prevention of constipation is a key nursing task; discussion with the stoma care nurse specialist regarding recommendations for diet and fibre supplements should be undertaken. The palliative care specialist may also be able to make other recommendations if normal dietary supplements are not tolerated well by the palliative care patient. The palliative care nurse or stoma care nurse specialist should be contacted if the problem becomes severe and requires more active intervention. Enemas are of limited use and a stoma will not retain suppositories.

Bleeding from the stoma is fairly common and can usually be stopped by applying pressure. If bleeding becomes a major problem it may be due to tumour infiltration of the stoma and local palliative radiotherapy or cryotherapy may need to be considered.

Nausea with or without vomiting is another common problem during the palliative care phase; whilst vomiting once or twice a day may be acceptable to many patients, continuous nausea will not be. It is important for the community nurse to identify the nature of the problem, what exacerbates the symptoms and what helps; whether the problem is transient or continuous; and whether the patient has any other symptoms that may identify the possible cause. Often nausea can be associated with drugs, the smell of food cooking and the sight of food. Vomiting may be associated with disease progression, for example obstruction or raised intercranial pressure, and may require more urgent intervention.

Food is often a key issue between the patient and their loved ones, as food is seen as sustaining life and 'if you don't eat you must be dying'. The community nurse's role is in educating the family to offer little and often, avoiding fried or grilled foods and to avoid very smelly foods, such as smoked fish. Using a microwave, extractor fan and shutting the door from the kitchen to the rest of the house can be helpful. The use of foods such as ginger biscuits and peppermint tea may reduce nausea, while some patients may opt for Earl Grey tea and a plain biscuit. Encouraging the patient to experiment with 'cures', as well as identifying causes of their nausea, is often preferable to adding another drug to the prescription sheet of the patient. However, ensuring the patient does not suffer undue symptoms for any length of time is of most importance, so careful monitoring and assessment must be given.

Fistulas and skin infiltration occur in about 3% of patients with advanced disease (Waller, 1996). Patients with gastrointestinal tumours and those who have received abdominal radiation are most at risk of fistula formation. Few complications cause as much distress to the patient and their loved ones as highly malodorous fungating lesions or high-output fistulas. Ostomy appliances are often of great benefit in collecting fluid and reducing odour. The range of paediatric appliances is more adaptable for small fistulas and the stoma care nurse specialist will be able to advise on skin care and the most appropriate appliance.

Fungating lesions are often caused by anaerobic organisms and may be effectively treated using metronidazole 0.8% topical gel. Charcoal dressings are very effective at absorbing odours from smelly wounds and have been utilised for some time. Other effective substances that have been identified are natural yoghurt, applied after the skin has been cleaned and dried, and honey, which may also help in wound healing. Aromatherapy also has a place in disguising the smell in the patient's room. Aromatherapy needs to be advised by a competent practitioner who can offer advice and ensure the aroma utilised is acceptable to the patient and appropriate for the problem. Local radiotherapy has been identified as useful especially when there is constant bleeding from the lesion. The palliative care nursing team will be able to advise on more difficult problems associated with larger fungating lesions.

Pain is the most feared symptom for the majority of patients and their families (Twycross, 1997). When considering the pain presentation in the palliative care patient it is worthwhile to consider Dame Cecily Saunders' concept of 'total pain' (Clark and Seymour, 1999). This is pain that is influenced by the physical, psychological, spiritual and social state of the patient. Often it is as important to sit and discuss the cause of the pain as it is to increase the analgesic dose. The most important role for the community nurse is the assessment of the pain and the pain management. It has been estimated that over 50% of patients in the palliative phase have poorly controlled pain. This is often due to poor assessment of the cause of the pain and the appropriateness of the analgesia being given (Hanks, 1995; Twycross, 1997). If it can be clearly identified, for example, that the patient is very anxious, the use of an anxiolytic drug such as Diazepam or Haloperidol may be far more appropriate in improving pain control than an increase in morphine (Twycross, 1995).

The use of pain assessment tools that give a constant picture of the patient's pain control are imperative. Ensuring the patient, or relatives, write down when the pain increases, any thoughts as to why the pain has increased and what the patient did to relieve the pain will give a more complete picture. This information can then be utilised to assess the appropriateness of the dosage of the opioids and any adjuvent drugs being utilised.

For most nurses, caring for a palliative or terminal patient who has uncontrolled pain is one of the most difficult scenarios. By undertaking a continuous and thorough assessment of the pain and the pain management this situation should be kept to a minimum. Utilising the palliative care nurse specialist or the hospice team for advice on pain management will always improve the outcome.

In some instances it is viewed as appropriate to utilise what could be considered as 'active' treatment for symptom management in the palliative care patient. This requires very careful planning, as the benefits of any treatment must be viewed in terms of quality of life. If the patient could potentially receive symptom relief from the use of surgery, radiotherapy or chemotherapy, the patient's physical state is appropriate to minimise morbidity and the patient wishes to undertake further treatment, then active treatment should always be viewed as an option. The patient must, however, be fully aware of the consequences of the treatment options and must also understand that while it is active treatment it is given to palliate not to cure. Patients often undertake further 'treatment' to please loved ones or as 'one last attempt at cure'. While the importance of hope must not be underestimated, realistic hope needs to be discussed. Often the patient will ask the community nurse or practice nurse for advice as to whether to proceed; they are also often the first to be informed when the patient has had enough. Acting as the patient's advocate is an important role and should be based on an understanding of the treatment options.

PALLIATIVE SURGERY

It is fair to say that many patients with cancer still present at an advanced stage. For example, advanced disease at presentation of colorectal cancer occurs in about 20% of patients. For palliative treatment surgery has a major role as part of a multiple modality approach. It has a role in 'inoperable' primary disease, local or regional recurrence, metastatic disease and intestinal obstruction. Intestinal obstruction is particularly common in ovarian cancer (25–40%) and colorectal cancer (10–15%) and less frequently in endometrial, bladder and prostate cancer.

Surgery should be considered in the management of every patient with intestinal obstruction because in many cases the obstruction may be due to a benign cause or a resectable new primary (Waller, 1996). Patients need to be identified as appropriate for surgery with a reasonable performance status (Table 5.2) and a reasonable gap since previous surgery. However, even with careful selection, surgical morbidity from faecal fistula, reobstruction, dehiscence and sepsis as well as surgical mortality remains high.

Table 5.2 WHO performance status

Grade 0	Normal activity
Grade 1	Ambulatory, can do light work
Grade 2	Bed or chair for up to 50% of waking hours, but self-caring
Grade 3	Bed or chair for more than 50% of waking hours, limited self-care
Grade 4	Confined to bed or chair, no self-care, completely disabled

As with all treatments the benefits and the wishes of the patient must be considered. To be told that you have cancer, that the outlook is extremely bleak and on top of all that you require a stoma can be devastating, (Randles 1998). This additional blow exacerbates fears of loss of control, loss of dignity and fears of rejection from family and friends. In recent years minimal access surgery has been shown to have the advantages of reduced hospital stay and quicker patient recovery. Other palliative surgery techniques have been developed, such as colonic stents, which will relieve obstruction and may be used with laser tumour ablation or radiotherapy. These may avoid the need for a stoma in some patients (Hershman, 1998).

Ileal conduits may have been formed previously for benign disease; it would be unusual to perform a palliative ileal conduit. Care for these patients is similar to that for any stoma patient, with advice from the specialist stoma care nurse if problems arise. A nephrostomy is more likely to be performed to relieve ureteric obstruction and requires careful handling to prevent it becoming dislodged, causing inconvenience to the patient.

Palliative surgery should be offered as part of a team approach to ensure optimal quality of life for the patient with incurable disease. However, if the patient has a relatively good quality of life and is in reasonable general health, then the use of surgery to relieve symptoms may be highly recommended. Some patients and professionals question the use of active treatment for the palliative patient. But who would not recommend the formation of an ostomy if it saved the patient from the pain, faecal vomiting and misery of obstruction (Doyle, 1996)?

CHEMOTHERAPY

The utilisation of modified chemotherapy and radiotherapy regimes can vastly improve the management of a range of symptoms.

Palliative chemotherapy may be given to patients with local or advanced disease in order to prolong life, control symptoms or improve quality of life; it is probably fair to say that most chemotherapy is palliative from the outset (Kaye, 1997). Cancers most commonly treated with palliative chemotherapy are colorectal, cervix, ovary and bladder, although as newer drugs are being utilised this list is growing. There has also been progress in the identification of drugs that have similar 'response' rates but reduced side effects, such as Tomudex (raltitrexed) for colorectal cancer.

When deciding to offer chemotherapy it must be remembered that given correctly it can be of great benefit in terms of prolonging life and/or symptom control. If given inappropriately it may hasten death and the toxicity can destroy any quality of life.

One of the most important issues is the careful selection of patients. Identification of the patient's performance status (see Table 5.2) is useful as patients with a poor performance are less likely to respond to treatment and are more likely to die from the toxicity. Another factor is bulk of disease, for example in ovarian cancer, when surgery for debulking may enhance the effectiveness of chemotherapy improving tumour shrinkage.

The key question that needs to be answered while the patient is undergoing treatment is, 'Does it make them feel better?' In a study by Slevin (1990) it was demonstrated that an individual's philosophy changes when in the palliative stage of life and that these individuals were prepared to accept treatment that offered little or no chance of benefit. It is important that the goals of treatment are clearly defined from the beginning, so that lack of response or discontinuation of treatment does not have a severe psychological impact on the patient.

Community nurses with a close relationship with the patient and an understanding of the potential benefits and disadvantages of chemotherapy can support the patient to make informed choices, at a time when the patient is vulnerable to pressure from professionals and families.

The drugs utilised are those that have been identified as demonstrating a response for a specific tumour; the tumour must therefore be chemosensitive. Investigations will be carried out prior to the commencement of treatment to assess the extent of the disease and the competence of the patient's liver and renal function, so that the drugs can be given safely. Monitoring investigations will continue during treatment to assess response to the chemotherapy and identify any potential toxic side effects, such as neutropenia.

Nausea is of concern as these patients may have already been nauseated due to the disease or morphine-based drugs. The more potent anti-emetic drugs have increased the range of palliative chemotherapy drugs that can now be utilised. Regular assessment to ensure that the patient is not suffering from nausea is important. Patients are sometimes reluctant to discuss their problems with the oncologist and chemotherapy specialist nurses for fear that they will stop 'treating'.

Another common side effect of both chemotherapy and radiotherapy is fatigue; patients will often need advice on how to maximise their energy levels and adapt their life style to ensure the quality of their life is maintained. It is important that any patient undergoing chemotherapy is carefully monitored to ensure that the potential toxicities from the drugs do not impact on the patient's quality of life.

PALLIATIVE RADIOTHERAPY

Radiation therapy has a role to play in controlling and preventing a range of symptoms. It is most frequently utilised to relieve pain caused by bone secondaries, which are particularly associated with pelvic tumours. Any tumour arising in the genitourinary or gastrointestinal tract is often amenable to irradiation, with a single fraction of radiation therapy often relieving pelvic and bone pain (Needham, 1997). Rectal pain, bleeding and discharge caused by inoperable or recurrent rectal carcinoma can often be palliated in 80–90% of patients using a short course of external beam radiotherapy. Some work is being undertaken to identify the potential of brachytherapy in local recurrent tumour. This is a form of radiotherapy in which the radioactive source is placed close to or inside the tumour.

Spinal cord compression is a palliative emergency, which can totally destroy the patient's quality of life. Early detection of the onset of spinal cord compression and rapid access to radiotherapy will improve response rates.

When offering palliative radiotherapy, side effects must always be kept to a minimum: the aim of palliative radiotherapy being symptom relief not tumour elimination. Shrinkage of the tumour is a common reaction to a dose of radiotherapy, which in itself may alleviate symptoms, although the response to the therapy may take as long as four weeks to manifest. Therefore patients with a limited life span may experience limited or no benefit (Campbell, 1998).

The commonest side effect associated with palliative radiotherapy is fatigue, which may continue for some time after treatment. Patients need to be aware that this is a side affect of the treatment and not an indication of disease progression. Another potential side effect is associated with abdominal radiotherapy when patients may have nausea, vomiting and diarrhoea. Dietetic advice and information is essential to ensure these symptoms do not distress the patient.

Skin toxicity may be a complication, although this is dose dependent and should not be a problem for patients receiving palliative doses. Patients should be advised not to use perfumed or scented products as these may react with the radiation resulting in erythema (Campbell, 1998). Assessment of skin integrity and signs of redness will enable early treatment to be initiated. Advice should be sought from the palliative care specialist nurse or the radiotherapy clinic nurse if this becomes problematic.

CONCLUSION

The community nurse has a key role in the delivery of palliative care for the patient with a life limiting disease. Ensuring that the patient has minimal symptoms and active management of symptoms involves close assessment and sound knowledge of appropriate treatments. Promoting open and complete communication between the patient, carers and the multiprofessional team will enable early identification of potential problems.

The patient with a stoma may have fewer problems in the terminal phase as they will not have the indignity of incontinence. Incontinence, particularly faecal incontinence, is often seen as indicative of a loss of dignity. Having to rely on loved ones to change the bed and being aware of making a mess is extremely distressing for the dying patient.

However, patients with a stoma need to have their care planned by the team to ensure the stoma management is maintained at an optimal level. Pro-active management is an integral part of the successful holistic approach to the delivery of effective palliative care and by utilising the specialist stoma care nurse and the specialist palliative care nurse this will ensure that all symptoms are managed effectively.

Learning outcomes

▸ The meaning of palliative care.

▸ The key issues in symptom management.

▸ The importance of assessment in care planning.

▸ The importance of a multiprofessional approach to palliative care.

▸ The importance of surgery, chemotherapy and radiotherapy in symptom management.

REFERENCES

Campbell, T., Farrell, W. (1998) Palliative radiotherapy for advanced cancer symptoms. *International Journal of Palliative Care;* 4: 6, 292–299.

Clark, D., Seymour, J. (1999) *Reflections on palliative care.* Buckingham: Open University Press.

Doyle, D. (1996) *Domiciliary Palliative Care: A Guide for the Primary Care Team.* Oxford: Oxford University Press.

Dunlop, R., Kaye, P. (1997) Palliative care – the next 10 years. In: Kaye, P. (ed.) *Tutorials in Palliative Medicine.* Northampton: EPL Publications.

Grande, G.E., Todd, C.J., Barclay, S.I.G. et al (1996) What terminally ill patients value in the support provided by GPs, district and Macmillan nurses. *International Journal of Palliative Care;* 2: 3.

Hanks, G. (1995) Problem areas in pain and symptom management in advanced cancer patients. *European Journal of Cancer;* 31a, 869–870.

Hershman, M., Rooney, P., Ramesh, S. (1998) Palliative surgery for colorectal cancer. *Palliative Care Today;* V11: 111, 18–19.

Ingham, J.M., Coyle, N. (1997) Teamwork in end-of-life care: a nurse–physician perspective on introducing physicians to palliative care concepts. In: Clark, D., Hockley, J., Ahmedzai, S. (eds.) *New Themes in Palliative Care*. Buckingham: Open University Press.

Jenkins, R. (1997) Nursing care. In: Kaye, P. (ed.) *Tutorials in Palliative Medicine*. Northampton: EPL Publications.

Needham, P. (1997) Palliative radiotherapy. In: Kaye, P. (ed.) *Tutorials in Palliative Medicine.* Northampton: EPL Publications.

Randles, J. (1998) The psychological problems of stoma patients. *Palliative Care Today;* V11: 111, 22–23.

Slevin, M.L., Stubbs, L., Plant, H.J. (1990) Attitudes to chemotherapy: comparing views of patients with cancer with those of doctors, nurses and general public. *British Medical Journal;* 300: 1458–60

Twycross, R. (1995) *Introducing Palliative Care*. Oxford: Radcliffe Medical Press.

Twycross, R. (1997) *Symptom Management in Advanced Cancer*. 2nd Edition. Oxford: Radcliffe Medical Press.

Waller, A., Caroline, N.L. (1996) *Handbook of Palliative Care in Cancer*. Oxford: Butterworth Heinemann.

World Health Authority (1990) *Cancer Pain Relief and Palliative Care*. Geneva: World Health Organisation.

6 Psychological aspects of stoma care

Craig A. White

It is not possible to provide nursing care to people who have stomas without having to consider the psychological impact of the surgery on their life. Stoma surgery involves significant changes in body form and functioning which are associated with increased self-care demands and involve adaptation in almost every life domain (Bekkers et al, 1997), and which can have a profound and lasting psychosocial impact. Patients often report concerns about appearance, smell, odour, relationships, sexual function and social functioning. In this chapter I will outline the main psychological issues which are relevant for the care of those who undergo surgery resulting in the formation of a stoma, with particular emphasis on psychological assessment and management. The importance of understanding psychological processes, which underpin adjustment to this form of surgery, will be highlighted throughout this chapter.

THE PROCESS OF PSYCHOLOGICAL ADJUSTMENT

The process of psychological adjustment to stoma surgery will differ between individual patients. However, there are common themes that occur in the psychological concerns of patients (White and Hunt, 1997). All patients will be concerned to varying degrees with their appearance and the day to day impact of the functional changes in their bowel or bladder functioning. For some people these concerns and issues will precipitate the signs and symptoms of a mental disorder that will require treatment. For others the surgery will cause problems that compromise their overall quality of life. However, there is also a sizeable proportion of patients for whom the surgery results in an improvement in mental health (Thomas et al, 1984) which may have been previously significantly compromised by the effects of a chronic medical problem, such as ulcerative colitis. A further group of patients may have psychological problems that relate to events that are separate from their illness and its surgical treatment. Examples of this might include a pre-existing relationship problem, social anxiety or an eating disorder. Significant psychological symptomatology following stoma surgery (irrespective of origins or preoperative psychological status) is experienced by approximately 18–26% of patients (Thomas et al, 1984; Wade, 1990; White and Unwin, 1998). These figures are of a similar magnitude to those for patients who have undergone other forms of major surgery and/or following the diagnosis of diseases such as cancer.

The factors associated with postoperative psychological problems can be thought of in terms of preoperative factors and postoperative factors. Patients with a past psychiatric history are at a greater risk of psychological problems following surgery (Thomas et al, 1987, Wade, 1990; White and Unwin, 1998) as are those patients who report lower levels of satisfaction with preoperative preparation (Follick et al, 1984; Thomas et al, 1987). Patients who are experiencing stoma related physical symptoms, such as leakage, peristomal skin problems or prolapse, are more likely to experience psychological symptoms (Thomas et al, 1987; Oberst and Scott, 1988; Wade, 1990; White and Unwin, 1988). Cognitive factors have also been shown to be associated with poorer psychological adjustment. White and Unwin (1998) found that patient beliefs about physical integrity, impact of the stoma on their lives and whether they felt they were in control of their bodies were significantly related to levels of psychological distress. Bekkers et al (1996) reported that patients with higher levels of stoma care self-efficacy (confidence in their abilities to care for their stoma) had higher levels of psychosocial adjustment in the first four postoperative months. They also investigated social self-efficacy (confidence with regard to social functioning with a stoma) and found that higher levels were associated with better psychosocial adjustment at both four months and 12 months postoperatively. Factors such as age, marital status, severity of illness, presurgical diagnosis, gender and type of stoma have not been shown to be related to psychosocial adjustment following this form of surgery (see White and Hunt, 1997 for review).

ASSESSMENT OF PSYCHOSOCIAL VARIABLES

Psychological concerns, problems and symptoms can present before, during and after surgical treatment. All nursing staff should be confident and competent with regard to the identification of common psychological concerns and screening for the presence of major psychological problems or disorders. The most common psychological disorders to present following stoma surgery are: adjustment disorders; anxiety disorders, such as panic disorder, generalised anxiety disorder and agoraphobia; major depressive disorder; and sexual dysfunction. There is an increasing amount of evidence which indicates that post traumatic stress disorder is prevalent to a significant degree among people who have had a life threatening illness such as cancer (Baider and de Nour, 1997). It is possible that some people will experience these symptoms postoperatively. There are also many people who will have symptoms which, although not present with sufficient frequency and intensity to warrant a formal diagnosis, will significantly compromise their overall psychological wellbeing and the quality of the social and sexual aspects of their lives (Bekkers et al, 1997). Nursing staff play a vital role in identifying the psychological needs of their patients and providing practical nursing care which is sensitive to these needs. This care should integrate psychosocial support and symptom screening with vigilance for the occurrence of psychological problems (Borwell, 1997). It can be helpful for nursing staff to have a good understanding of the main signs and symptoms of the common psychological disorders which can occur and, importantly, the sorts of screening questions which can be used to elicit these symptoms (Table 6.1).

Many of the concerns which people with a stoma have are often discussed in term of body image problems. Fisher (1990) argues that 'one also needs to recognise that there are indeed quite different and perhaps largely independent dimensions represented under the rough rubric of 'body image". There is no such entity as 'The Body Image'. The term is often used to refer to different components of the same construct by different researchers and clinicians. A detailed review of the main psychological dimensions of body image is outside the scope of this chapter. Recent evidence suggests that body image should be regarded as a cognitive structure which represents the sum of previous appearance-related experiences and which serves as a template to direct attention, influence encoding and interpretation and facilitate recall of information regarding self-evaluative information about one's appearance. Price (1998) offers a useful introduction to some of these issues from a nursing perspective.

Table 6.1 Main symptoms of common psychological disorders (with screening questions)

Psychological disorder	Main symptoms	Screening questions
Panic Disorder	Recurrent panic attacks	Do you ever get a sudden rush of fear or discomfort?
	Concern about more attacks	
		Is that accompanied by physical sensations?
	Worry about losing control	
	Changed behaviour related to attacks	What is the worse thing that could happen when this is going on?
		Do you do anything differently to cope with these attacks?
Major Depressive Disorder	Depressed mood	How have you been feeling in your spirits?
	Diminished interest in activities	
	Weight loss or appetite change	Do you get the same amount of enjoyment from what you do?
	Sleep problems	
	Agitation	How do you feel about yourself compared to other people?
	Loss of energy	
	Feeling worthless or guilty	Do you ever feel that life is not worth living?
	Recurrent thoughts of death or suicide	
Generalised Anxiety Disorder	Excessive worry and anxiety most days for at least six months	Are you ever troubled by worrying thoughts that go round and round in your head?
	Difficult to control the worry	
	Associated with restlessness, fatigue, irritability, muscle tension, sleep problems or concentration problems	Are you able to control these worrying thoughts?

Psychological disorder	Main symptoms	Screening questions
Social Phobia	Persistent fear of one or more social/performance situations	How do you feel about being in social situations?
	Anxious about acting in humiliating or embarrassing way	Do you ever worry about being embarrassed or making a fool of yourself?
	Exposure to situation almost always results in anxiety	When you are not in the situation how do you think and feel?
	Recognises fear is excessive	
	Avoids situations or endures with distress	
Post Traumatic Stress Disorder	Experience of event involving actual/threatened death or injury	Does the event ever come back to your mind when you don't want it to?
	Intensely fearful, helpless or terrified	How do you feel when you are reminded of the event?
	Recurrent distressing thoughts, images or nightmares of event	Do you do anything to avoid things about the event?
	Intense physical and psychological distress when reminded of event	Are you bothered by being on edge or very jumpy?
	Effort to avoid reminders of event	
	Diminished interest in activities	
	Hypervigilance or exaggerated startle response	
	Irritability or outbursts of anger	

Psychological signs, symptoms, problems and concerns are often not identified by healthcare staff (Bridges and Goldberg, 1984; Feldman et al, 1987; Mayou and Hawton, 1986). There are many potential reasons for this, including concern that it will be difficult to manage problems once they are elicited, that this will be emotionally overwhelming and/or that there is not enough time to assess psychological aspects of personal experiences (Faulkner and Maguire, 1994). Nurses should routinely screen for the most commonly occurring psychosocial concerns (Table 6.2). It is often assumed that if a concern is important enough then a patient will mention it. This is not always the case – patients may actively avoid mentioning certain concerns for fear that it is not appropriate or that it will result in a waste of a busy staff member's time. It has also been suggested that the manner in which outpatient consultations are organised may not always be conducive to the disclosure of concerns (Rubin and Devlin, 1987).

Table 6.2 Main psychosocial concerns of stoma patients

Not being complete as a person
General impact of stoma on life (e.g. 'rules my life')
Feeling in control of body
Whether other people will hear or smell stoma
Influence on intimacy and sexual function
Being able to deal with stoma care

Self-report questionnaires can be used as part of the process of determining a patient's precise psychological needs, to monitor changes in symptoms over time and, in some situations, to evaluate responses to a nursing intervention. The Stoma Cognitions Questionnaire (White and Unwin, 1998) measures the degree to which patients agree or disagree with statements about their stoma. This measure can complement clinical interviewing and be a useful way of eliciting concerns about life with a stoma. The Stoma Self-Efficacy Scale (Bekkers et al, 1996) is particularly useful for the assessment of confidence in ability to manage the demands of the stoma care routine (stoma care self-efficacy) and the ability to manage the social impact of living with a stoma (social self-efficacy). The Hospital Anxiety and Depression (HAD) Scale (Zigmond and Snaith, 1983) is a well-known measure most often used as a screening measure for symptoms. It has often been included in psychosocial research as an outcome measure. The usefulness of the HAD Scale has recently been questioned and the 12 item version of the General Health Questionnaire (Goldberg, 1992) has been cited a better measure to use for screening for psychological symptoms (Hall et al, 1999).

It has been suggested that all patients who have had surgery resulting in the formation of a stoma should be screened for the presence of psychological symptoms at three months postoperatively (Thomas et al, 1987). This could be easily achieved if a self-report measure was routinely incorporated into the postoperative screening process. Indeed, the administration of a measure could be incorporated into assessment protocols to monitor psychological health at preoperative, predischarge and postoperative stages. There is a common misconception that such routine screening would involve a huge amount of additional human resources and time. However, the implementation of this would be unlikely to involve significant resources beyond the purchase of individual questionnaires, most of which take less than 10 minutes to complete and score. There would be resource implications for how the psychosocial needs identified at screening were addressed. For this reason, any new screening measures implemented as part of routine care should be accompanied by an audit of service responses to identified needs. This means that gaps in psychological care services can be minimised by planning service developments. In many surgical services it is probably not practical for this type of screening to be incorporated into routine practice for every patient. It is more likely that regular screening could be carried out for patients who have risk factors for psychosocial problems.

MANAGEMENT OF PSYCHOLOGICAL HEALTH

The primary aim of psychosocially sensitive assessments is to identify psychological concerns, issues and problems. Assessment is a crucial first stage, but to complete the process nursing staff will then need to respond to these in an appropriate manner. There are many strategies that can be implemented in the management of psychosocial aspects of patient care. These include:

- the provision of psychosocial support via the implementation of listening and counselling skills;

- nursing intervention to address a physical problem which is compromising psychological health (for example leakage or odour);

- monitoring of psychological symptoms;

- referral to a specialist in mental health;

- the implementation of time limited strategies to address concerns and promote optimal wellbeing.

Staff concerns about not knowing what to do when issues are identified can significantly contribute to problems with their identification. It is therefore highly desirable that nurses have a clear idea of the management options that they have in this area.

Prevention

Factors shown to be associated with psychological problems after stoma surgery can form the basis of efforts aimed at prevention and/or early identification of those at risk. In a substantial proportion of cases patients will know in advance that they are to have stoma surgery. A preoperative assessment of psychological status should aim to determine if the patient has any ongoing psychological problems and should screen for the presence of any risk factors that may place them at increased risk after surgery. The preparation of a psychologically sensitive care plan should always be a priority. This is not always easy, as there are few models to assist with identifying optimal models of psychological care delivery. The following table contains examples of some typical aims appearing in a psychologically sensitive care plan.

Table 6.3 Examples of psychologically oriented components of nursing care plans

To prepare patient for surgery by providing information on procedural and sensory aspects

To determine if any risk factors for psychological problems are present

To promote greater stoma care self-efficacy

To assess patient satisfaction with information

To enhance satisfaction with information

To enable patient to break down goal of returning to work into smaller steps

To monitor psychological symptoms at outpatient appointment

To inform colleagues in hospital/community of risk factors for psychological problems

Preparation for surgery (including information provision)

Psychological preparation for surgical procedures has been shown to result in numerous psychological and physical health benefits (Johnston and Vogele, 1993) and should be an integral part of the preparatory work which nurses might undertake before someone is admitted for stoma surgery (Borwell, 1997; Black, 1998). It is generally accepted that such preparatory work should cover what is going to happen before, during and after surgery (procedural information) and how they will feel throughout the process (sensory information). There are many information booklets available for patients that explain what stoma surgery involves and aspects of self-care routines.

Efforts should be made to enhance an individual patient's satisfaction with the information that they have been given as this may confer a prophylactic effect psychologically. The most sensible first steps are to establish what is already known and then to ensure that the patient is provided with the information that they want. They should be encouraged to consider the potential impact of receiving information (they may not have thought about how they will feel if the information they get differs from hopes or expectations). Information needs should always be assessed individually. Patients can be asked to list the questions which they have and, when practical, to take these to a subsequent appointment. Given the established links which exist between preoperative information provision and satisfaction, it is imperative that people are asked first to report how satisfied they are with the information that they have been provided with and second, what would need to happen for them to be more satisfied. Information provision aimed at enhancing satisfaction can then take place. Subsequent satisfaction checks can be done to determine whether the information has had the desired enhancing effects. The information provided should be given with reference to the established principles for providing information, which are outlined later in this chapter.

Nurse: Dr Matthews told me that you have your date to go for the operation. I wondered if I could ask you some questions about this to see if there are any ways that we can help you before and after this surgery.

Patient: I see.

Nurse: What have you been told about what is going to happen?

(Nurse determines what patient knows about their problem.)

Patient: Well I know I have this growth; a tumour which they need to take out. And something about a bag that I'll have. I just want it out of me, to get rid of it.

Nurse: So you know that you have a tumour that the surgeon is going to remove and that after the operation you'll have a bag? Is there anything else that you've been told about what's going to happen?

Patient: No, just that I'll be in for about 10 days.

Nurse: How satisfied would you say you are with the information that you have so far? Think of this on a scale from 0 to 100, where zero means not at all satisfied and one hundred is the most satisfied you could be.

Patient: Can I give it any score? Well, about 20... yes, 20.

Nurse: I want you to be as satisfied as you possibly can be. Think about what information you would need for that score to be higher. Can you tell me what you would need to know for the satisfaction to go up?

The satisfaction rating should be determined again and, if necessary, the steps repeated.

There are some rules that should be followed when providing information for patients. This advice is based on many years of research by psychologists about which information provision strategies promote enhanced recall, compliance and satisfaction, and quicker recovery from illness (Ley and Llewelyn, 1995). It is advisable to make sure that important information is given first of all. This is more likely to be recalled because of the 'primacy effect'. Stressing the importance of information, explicitly categorising the information and repeating the categories as information giving progresses will increase recall. Repetition of material increases recall and has beneficial effects on satisfaction.

This is an example of how explicit categorisation can be used:

There are three things that you might find it helpful to know about the bags. First, what they are for, second how you will learn to deal with your own bag and third what arrangements there will be for helping you with this. First, what the bag is for. It is a way of collecting the waste material that cannot escape in the usual way because part of your bowel is going to be removed by the surgeons...

Increasing self-efficacy

Some patients will have difficulty mastering the skills involved in a stoma care routine. These skill acquisition difficulties may relate to a global lack of confidence in their ability to manage anything in their lives, may be confined to the tasks involved or to specific situations or may be attributable to a lack of information on what to do. There are, of course, factors associated with problems such as depression (that is, lack of motivation) and dementia (that is, impaired memory and praxis) which can make assimilation of the skills difficult.

The choice of nursing intervention in these cases will depend on the main factor contributing to the problem. Most psychosocial problems in stoma care can be conceptualised as related in some way to a lack of self-efficacy in the component parts of the stoma care routine (even if they are only a secondary consequence of another problem). As a result, in most cases enhancing stoma care self-efficacy will lead to an improvement in psychosocial functioning. An example of this would be social anxiety mediated by a lack of confidence that the appliance has been securely attached. Addressing patient confidence in this aspect of their self-care should address their social anxiety.

The promotion of self-efficacy can be achieved if patients are supported to learn each component part of their stoma care routine in isolation, repeatedly and until they notice changes in their confidence levels. These changes can be monitored using a confidence diary. This will provide the patient with information on their progress and/or the nurse with information on where they may be struggling. It can be reinforcing for patients to monitor the changes in their confidence levels. White (1997) has suggested how the components of changing a stoma care appliance can be broken down and data collected on confidence ratings as postoperative recovery progresses (Table 6.4). Patients may also find it easier to learn skills if they are demonstrated first by someone else (for example, by using a video or live demonstration) and if they learn them in a similar setting to that in which they have to carry them out.

Table 6.4 Confidence diary

Date:	November 10 1998
Location:	Ward 1B
Postoperative days:	10
Confidence scale:	0 10 20 30 40 50 60 70 80 90 100
	Not at all Very
	confident confident

Activity	Confidence rating (0–100)
Removing appliance from skin	34
Emptying the appliance	60
Washing/drying the stoma site	30
Measuring stoma size	34
Putting appliance on	10
Disposal of used appliance	25

Note: Component activities will differ according to stoma care routine

Many patients become concerned about their first encounters with situations that previously would not have caused them any problems. Much of the rehabilitation process following surgery is characterised by enabling people to tackle problems in manageable steps at a pace that suits the overall context of their postoperative recovery. Clinical psychologists often use a treatment technique called graded exposure to tackle avoidance mediated by anxiety. This can be a useful way to think of helping people tackle the small steps they will need to take to make a full recovery in separate life domains. The technique consists of two components: first, breaking a larger goal or task into as many smaller steps as possible, and then ranking these steps according to degree of difficulty, anxiety, pain and so on (Table 6.5). Each small step can be tackled in increasing order of difficulty until the patient has mastered the final step. Problems and setbacks can be dealt with by suggesting that the patient resumes at an earlier stage or that they insert a smaller leap from one step to the next.

Table 6.5 Graded exposure technique

Final goal: Go to Sheila's coffee morning

Step	Description	*Anxiety rating (0–10)*		
		predicted	actual	date(s)
1	Go into corner shop	6	4	4 June
		5	3	5 June
2	Visit Doreen	8	4	6 June
3	Go to post office	7	3	8 June
		5	3	9 June
4	Go to supermarket	4	2	9 June
		4	2	10 June
5	Go to Sheila's coffee morning	5	1	13 June

Reviewing and responding to negative thinking

Many psychological problems are characterised by negative thinking patterns. It is these thoughts which are often key maintaining factors for serious and more clinically significant problems with depression and anxiety. In such circumstances it is unlikely that simple advice on how to review and respond to thinking will have lasting effects (indeed, to provide only advice would be inappropriate). However, patients with less serious problems relating to anxiety and low mood may find it helpful to think about the way in which their thinking is influencing their psychosocial adjustment to surgery. Patients can be helped to identify their thoughts and evaluate them to see if there are more helpful alternatives. They should be advised to pay attention to what is going through their minds when they notice a change in their feelings (for example, a dip in their mood or a surge in anxiety). When they have identified some of the thoughts which they are having they can try to look for thinking biases or come up with alternatives by asking themselves a series of questions designed to shift their perspective or promote more helpful alternatives. By asking a series of simple questions when there is a mood change, thoughts can be identified. The evaluation of thoughts can be facilitated by reviewing common thinking biases and by asking another series of simple questions to facilitate a shift in perspective. Further details on the basic elements of this strategy can be found in White (1997) and Leahy (1997).

Table 6.6 Reviewing and responding to negative thinking

A Questions for identifying problem thoughts

1 What was going through my mind just as I started to have this problem mood?

2 What does this situation mean to me? What does this situation say about me?

3 What is the worst thing that could happen in this situation?

4 What have I just been thinking about?

5 What do I guess that I was thinking about just then?

B Common thinking biases

Problem thoughts are often the result of biases or distortions in thinking. These biases or distortions have special names. When you come to change problem thoughts it can be helpful to look for these biases. Some of the common biases are described below.

All-or-nothing thinking

Seeing things in black-and-white categories – either everything is going well or it is a complete disaster.

Over-generalisation

Seeing a single event as part of a never-ending pattern of events or generalising from one isolated event to the rest of our lives.

Mental filter

Picking out a single negative detail and focusing on it exclusively.

Discounting the positive

Saying that positive experiences don't count.

Jumping to conclusions

Drawing conclusions when there are no facts to support your conclusion. 'Mind-reading' is an example of this – you make predictions about what other people think as if you had mind-reading abilities. 'Fortune-telling' is another bias that involves jumping to conclusions. This involves predicting that something won't work out. You think things as if you can really see into the future.

Magnification

Exaggerating the importance of your difficulties and problems, and minimising your abilities to cope and your positive qualities.

Emotional reasoning

Assuming that your negative feelings are a reflection of the way that things really are.

Personalisation
Holding yourself personally responsible for an event that is not entirely under your control.

C   Questions for changing problem thoughts
1   What experiences have I had which show me that this thought is not completely true all the time?
2   If I were trying to help someone I cared about to feel better when they had this thought, what would I tell them?
3   What advice might someone I cared about give to me if they knew that I was thinking about things in this way? Would they agree with me? If not, why not?
4   When I am not experiencing this problem mood, how would I think about things?
5   What have I learned from previous events or experiences in my life which might help me to cope with this problem thought?
6   Is my problem thought an example of a thinking bias? If so, which one is it?
7   What is the evidence to support this thought? What is the evidence against this thought?
8   What is the worst thing that could happen? Could I live through and cope with this?
9   What is the best thing that could happen? What is the most realistic outcome?
10 What would be the effect of changing this problem thought? What can I do now?

Case management role

In order to manage psychosocial aspects of stoma surgery nursing staff need to:

- be confident about the processes of case management;

- know which specialist colleagues they can refer patients to;

- understand the nature of some of the interventions that may be recommended.

There are times when it may be necessary to make a referral to a clinical psychologist or psychiatrist for specialist opinion on a patient's psychological problems. Patients will often be concerned about issues such as madness and/or their physical problems not being taken seriously when referral is suggested. Nurses should be confident in how they can explain such a referral as a positive step in a patient's care. Retaining involvement with a patient after such a referral has been made is often helpful in terms of addressing concerns that may emerge about referral, and monitoring fluctuations in their symptoms. Liaison between mental health professionals and nurses before referral can be helpful as this can inform the process of case management. The sorts of questions that could be asked at this stage are outlined in the following table.

Table 6.7 Questions to ask mental health professionals

Are there things that I could be doing to help this patient with their problems until they are seen?

What would be signs that they are getting worse?

Is there any information that you could give me that you think would help them?

Are there any treatments/strategies that might help while they are waiting to see you?

Under what circumstances should I contact you again for further advice?

In some circumstances, it will not be clear whether a patient's problems are sufficiently severe to warrant referral to a specialist, such as a clinical psychologist or psychiatrist. Most clinical psychologists and psychiatrists will not mind being telephoned for advice on the management of a patient problem or to discuss whether a referral is appropriate or not. Many departments have arrangements for a member of staff to be available to advise colleagues. Most hospitals will also have some form of emergency rota for mental health problems (usually staffed by junior doctors undertaking training in psychiatry but sometimes by others, such as clinical psychologists and community psychiatric nurses). Early liaison between nurses and mental health colleagues is often essential, as there can be waiting lists for outpatient appointments with clinical psychologists and psychiatrists. In some cases, mental health professionals may make suggestions for new management strategies or how nursing colleagues can become involved in the care they are providing. In the case of drug treatments this may be monitoring patient responses or providing reinforcing advice on medication side effects. In the case of psychological treatment this could be collaborating with the specialist regarding the main elements of a treatment, such as increasing daily activity levels and/or keeping a diary of negative thoughts at times of lowered mood.

There are various interventions that might be recommended for patients with psychological problems. It can be helpful to know about these treatments – it could assist with decision-making about which professional to refer to (most UK clinical psychologists have training in cognitive behavioural therapies). It can also be helpful in explaining to patients what these treatments involve and/or in understanding what a patient will be exposed to if they experience various types of interventions. Cognitive behavioural therapy (CBT) is based on the view that our thoughts and beliefs have a significant influence on behaviours, emotions and physical reactions to life events and situations. It is a short-term, problem-oriented approach which aims to enable patients to identify, evaluate and change the unhelpful thoughts, beliefs and behaviours which are maintaining their psychological problems. CBT is the treatment of choice for anxiety disorders such as panic disorder, obsessive compulsive disorder, specific phobia and generalised anxiety disorder and has an important role in the management of depressive disorders, chronic pain problems and post traumatic stress disorder (Enright, 1997).

The other commonly available type of psychological treatment available on the NHS is psychodynamic psychotherapy. This type of treatment is usually of longer duration than CBT and is focused more on early relationships and conflicts. It is particularly suitable for personality problems and severe interpersonal and social problems.

Antidepressant drugs are often prescribed (alone or in conjunction with psychological approaches to treatment). These drugs are not addictive and often need to be taken for between two and four weeks before any symptomatic improvements are noticed. They also need to be taken for some time after the patient has improved as this protects against depressive recurrence and relapse. Anxiolytic (or anti-anxiety) drugs and hypnotic (sleep-inducing) drugs are not prescribed in the way that they used to be because of the potential for dependence. They can be helpful for short-term use, but there are many effective cognitive and behavioural strategies for the management of anxiety and sleep problems.

Troubleshooting

Undertaking assessment and management of psychosocial aspects following stoma surgery can mean that nursing staff will have to encounter difficult situations. Examples of this include times when someone refuses to talk about how they feel or where a patient says that everything is fine but the nurse suspects that this may not be the case.

There may also be times when patients make unreasonable demands on nursing staff and when nurses feel overwhelmed by patient feelings and problems. Although these are difficult to manage, there are some general guidelines that can help staff respond to them with confidence.

When patients refuse to talk about how they are feeling this should be acknowledged and they should be told that there will be someone to listen to them when they feel able to talk. It is helpful to offer the patient an explanation about why they might be finding it difficult to talk (for example, because of fears of powerful emotions) and to make the suggestion that not talking may be making things worse for them. In some circumstances, patient refusal to speak in this manner could be part of a serious mental illness that needs an urgent specialist opinion. In such circumstances the person is likely to demonstrate other signs and symptoms such as crying or unusual behaviours. When a nurse suspects problems that the patient denies, she should endeavour to summarise what she has heard the patient say and to follow this with a summary of her concerns. Patients presenting in this way can also be given information on how to access someone if they become aware of problems and/or want someone to talk to at some future time. Attempts to persuade the patient that things are not fine do not usually work and can alienate the patient. Those who feel confidence in their counselling skills can sometimes attempt gentle questioning about discrepancies between nurse and patient perspectives. For example: 'You said that you've had no problems since I last saw you. One of the nurses on the ward has been worried about some of the things you've said about your feelings. Do you know what she's been concerned about?'

There are times when patients will make unreasonable demands on staff skills and time. They may ask for secrets to be kept or make demands that the nurse deal with all their physical needs, social problems and psychological problems. It is important for staff to develop the confidence to define the limits of their expertise and role (however much this appears to conflict with the view that the nurse should be a universal solver of all problems). Clearly outlining the boundaries of involvement is crucial in addressing unreasonable demands. Talking with people about their psychological needs is often emotionally demanding, especially when nurses may be experiencing psychological concerns or problems in their own lives. Regular access to peer support and nursing supervision are crucial if staff are to be able to develop and enhance the quality of the psychological care they provide.

CONCLUSION

The provision of nursing care for those with a stoma is an inherently psychological process. Many of the concerns people have are psychological in nature and a substantial number of people will struggle with problems related to anxiety and depression. Nurses have a vital role in preventing, identifying and managing psychological concerns, problems, issues and disorders. Psychological wellbeing can be enhanced by:

- preparing people for surgery;

- providing information that is sensitive to need;

- promoting confidence in the stoma care routine and the gradual steps involved in recovery;

- providing advice on how to tackle negative thinking patterns;

- ensuring appropriate and timely referral for specialist advice and treatment when this is warranted.

Nurses also need to ensure they have access to supervision and advice regarding these aspects of their work as assessment and management of psychosocial issues can be challenging.

REFERENCES

Baider, L. de Nour, A. (1997) Psychological distress and intrusive thoughts in cancer patients. *Journal of Mental and Nervous Diseases;* 185: 5, 346–348.

Bekkers, N.J.T.M., van Knippenberg, F.C.E., van den Borne, H.W. et al (1996) Prospect of evaluation of psychosocial adaptation to stoma surgery: the role of self-efficacy. *Psychosomatic Medicine;* 58, 183–191.

Bekkers, N.J.T.M., van Knippenberg, F.C.E., van Dulmen, A.N. et al (1997) Survival and psychosocial adjustment to stoma surgery and non-stoma bowel resection: a four year follow-up. *Journal of Psychosomatic Research;* 42: 3, 235–244.

Black, P.K. (1998) Colostomy. *Professional Nurse;* 13, 851–857.

Borwell, B. (1997) Psychological considerations of stoma care nursing. *Nursing Standard;* 11: 48, 49–55.

Bridges, K.W., Goldberg, D.P. (1984) Psychiatric illness in in-patients with neurological disorders: patients' views on discussion of emotional problems with neurologists. *British Medical Journal;* 286, 656–658.

Enright, S.J. (1997) Cognitive behaviour therapy – clinical applications. *British Medical Journal*; 314, 1811–1816

Faulkener, A., Maguire, P. (1994) *Talking to Cancer Patients and Their Relatives*. Oxford: Oxford Medical.

Feldman, E., Mayou R, Hawton, K. et al (1987) Psychiatric disorder in medical inpatients. *Quarterly Journal of Medicine*; 63, 405–412.

Fisher, S. (1990) The evolution of psychological concepts about the body. In: Cash, T.F., Pruzinsky, T. (eds.) *Body Images: Development Deviance and Change*. New York: Guildford Press.

Follick, M.J., Smith, T.W., Turk, D.C. (1984) Psychosocial adjustment following ostomy. *Health Psychology*; 3, 505–517.

Goldberg, D. (1992) *General Health Questionnaire (GHQ–12)*. Windsor: NFER Nelson.

Hall, A., Hern R.A., Fallowfield, L. (1999) Are we using appropriate self report questionnaires for detecting anxiety and depression in women with early breast cancer? *European Journal of Cancer*; 15, 79–85.

Johnston, M., Vogele, C. (1993) Benefits of psychological preparation for surgery: a meta-analysis. *Annals of Behavioral Medicine*; 15, 245–256.

Leahy, R. (1997) *Cognitive Therapy: Basic Principles and Applications*. New Jersey: Jason Aronson Inc.

Ley, P., Llewelyn, S. (1995) Improving patients' understanding, recall, satisfaction and compliance. In: Broome, A., Llewelyn, S. (eds.) *Health Psychology: Processes and Applications* (2nd edition). London: Chapman and Hall.

Mayou, R.A., Hawton, K.E. (1986) Psychiatric disorders in the general hospital. *British Journal of Psychiatry*; 149, 172–190.

Oberst, M.T., Scott, D.W. (1988) Postdischarge distress in surgically treated cancer patients and their spouses. *Research in Nursing and Health*; 11, 223–233.

Price, B. (1998) Cancer: altered body image. *Nursing Standard*; 12, 49–55.

Rubin, G.P., Devlin, H.B. (1987) The quality of life with a stoma. *British Journal of Hospital Medicine*; 38, 300–306.

Thomas, C., Madden, F., Jehu, D. (1984) Psychosocial morbidity in the first three months following stoma surgery. *Journal of Psychosomatic Research*; 28, 251–257.

Thomas, C., Madden, F., Jehu, D. (1987) Psychological effects of stomas – II. Factors influencing outcome. *Journal of Psychosomatic Research;* 31, 317–323.

Wade, B.E. (1990) Colostomy patients: psychological adjustment at 10 weeks and one year after surgery in districts which employed stoma-care nurses and districts which did not. *Journal of Advanced Nursing;* 15, 1297–1304.

White, C.A., Hunt, J.C. (1997) Psychological factors in postoperative adjustment to stoma surgery. *Annals of the Royal College of Surgeons;* 3–7.

White, C.A., Unwin, J.C. (1998) Postoperative adjustment to surgery resulting in the formation of a stoma: the importance of stoma-related cognitions. *British Journal of Health for Psychology;* 3, 85–93.

White, C.A. (1997) *Living With a Stoma: A Practical Guide to Coping With Colostomy, Ileostomy or Urostomy.* London: Sheldon Press.

Zigmond, A.S., Snaith, R.P. (1983) The hospital anxiety and depression scale. *Acta Psychiatrica Scandinavia;* 67, 361–370.

FURTHER READING

Maguire, P., Haddad (1996) Psychological reactions to physical illness. In: Creed, F., Guthrie, E. (eds.). *Seminars in Liaison Psychiatry.* London: Gaskell Press.

This chapter, although written for trainee psychiatrists and medical students, provides a general introduction to the many issues that are relevant to the assessment and management of psychosocial aspects of medicine and surgery.

White, C.A. (1997) *Living with a Stoma: A Guide to Coping with Colostomy, Ileostomy or Urostomy.* London: Sheldon Press

This book is a practical guide to psychosocial aspects of stoma surgery. It is based on available psychosocial research and aims to promote knowledge and confidence and enable people to take steps to enhance their lives following surgery.

Leahy, R. (1997) *Cognitive Therapy: Basic Principles and Applications.* New Jersey: Jason Aronson Inc.

This book is an excellent introduction to cognitive therapy for beginners. It outlines the main applications and is illustrated with examples from clinical practice.

7 Sexuality and stoma care

Barbara Borwell

The aim of this chapter is to educate nurses on the effects stoma surgery may have on a person's sexuality.

DEFINITION OF SEXUALITY

Human sexuality is a complex issue and plays an important and integral part in our personalities, woven into the physical, social, psychological, cultural and spiritual aspects of our lives, and having an influence on every individual. Sexuality or sexual health has been defined by the World Health Organisation (1975) as 'the integration of the somatic, emotional, intellectual and social aspects of sexual being in ways that are positively enriching and that enhance personality, communication and love'. Sexuality is more than the act of sex; it is concerned with relationships and feelings about oneself and others. These in turn have an effect on self-esteem and self-worth. Sexual activity like any other lifestyle activity is variable; knowledge of the degree and desire for sexual activity is an important indicator for consideration when undertaking the initial nursing assessment.

Major changes in sexual role and function are experienced by patients who have undergone stoma surgery, in spite of the sphincter saving surgical techniques and moves towards continent procedures. Although many patients are effectively treated, sexual functioning morbidity remains a probable area of life disruption. Patients with a stoma have not only lost the means of normal elimination but, in addition, are left with abdominal scars and a protruding appendage on their abdomen. These threats, which can have a devastating effect on the mind as well as the body, varying with intensity and duration, are now recognised in nursing as quality of life issues.

For nurses to understand and recognise any changes in an individual's sexual role and function it is necessary to be familiar with the anatomy and physiology of the male and female reproductive organs, and have an awareness of those body parts which are potential sources of sexual pleasure.

FEMALE ANATOMY

External genitalia is the collective name for the vulva and includes the outer lips (labia majora), inner lips (labia minora), clitoris and vaginal orifice. These lie within the pelvic region. The urethra and anus are associated structures.

The introitus, or vaginal orifice, forms the entrance to the vagina and lies between the urethral opening and the anus. Inside the vagina and partly covering the opening lies a fine membrane known as the hymen.

The clitoris, which corresponds to the penis in the male as a source of sexual sensations, is about the size of a pea, and consists of elongated structures of erectile tissue attached to the pelvic bone. It lies at the top of the vulva, above the urethra opening, covered by a hood-like structure, which forms part of the labia. The glans clitoris, which is covered with a cap of skin, is made up of highly sensitive, vascular tissue.

The labia majora are two large folds of skin, filled with fibrous tissue and fat. Lying between the labia majora are two further thin folds of skin which are the labia minora. Together they form a boundary to the vulva, offering protection to the genitalia. Anteriorly they divide around the clitoris to form the prepuce and frenulum; posteriorly, the two are fused together to form the fouchette. The urethral and vaginal orifices are situated in the vestibule, which is the space adjacent to the labia minora.

Internal genitalia is the collective name given to the vagina, cervix, uterus, ovaries and Fallopian tubes.

The vagina is a hollow fibromuscular tube attaching the vulva to the uterus. It is this space which receives the penis in copulation. Lined with mucus membrane it is mainly without nerve endings and does not contain any glands. There is a proposed region in the front wall of the vagina, the Grafenberg spot or 'G' spot which is thought to have a high degree of erotic sensitivity. During sexual arousal, secretions that do occur are from the greater vestibular or cervical glands situated near the vaginal orifice. The vagina maintains a pH between 4.9 and 3.5 to minimise infection being introduced from the perineum, the hairless area of skin between the vagina and anus.

The uterus, a pear shaped hollow muscular organ, is situated in the pelvic cavity lying between the bladder and rectum. The flattened body of the uterus is situated over the bladder, with the neck of uterus connecting to the cervix, which protrudes through the anterior wall of the vagina, opening into the external Os. Anatomically the uterus consists of three layers: the outer wall – the perimetrium; a middle or muscular layer – the myometrium; and an inner layer or lining – the endometrium. Oestrogen and progesterone hormones secreted by the endocrine system are responsible for changes which occur in the endometrium during the menstrual cycle.

The two ovaries situated on either side of the uterus in the lower abdomen are the female sex glands that store ova and, in the menstrual cycle, produce hormones. Ova are conveyed by peristalsis down the Fallopian tubes, which are situated on either side of the ovary, into the uterus.

The female genital area receives its arterial blood supply from branches of the internal pudendal arteries, which branch from the external pudendal arteries maintained from the external iliac arteries. A network formed from branches of the uterine and vaginal arteries service the vagina. A large venous network connects into the internal iliac vein providing venous drainage to the area. Superficial and deep vaginal glands are responsible for lymph drainage from the vulva and vagina. The autonomic nervous system supplies the uterus and vagina, whereas the genitalia are supplied via the pudendal nerve (Gregory, 1997).

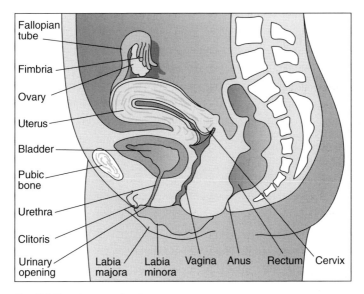

Fig 7.1 Female reproductive system

MALE ANATOMY

The external male genital organs are more visible and consist of the penis and scrotum, which contain further sub-structures.

Formation of the penis is primarily by three parallel cylinders, root and body is by the corpora cavernosa, a pair of cylinders made from tough fibrous tissue, and the tunica albuginea, filled with erectile tissue, which fills with blood during erection. The mechanism for erection is dependent on the structure of this tissue (Bancroft, 1989). The corpora cavernosa extend laterally into the body of the penis where they are attached to the pelvic bone. The corpus spongiosum lies along the underside of the penis between the corpora cavernosa, and contains the urethra, expanding at the distal end into a triangular tip, to form the glans penis. In uncircumcised males the prepuce or foreskin covers this. Blood supply is via branches of the internal pudendal arteries that feed into the deep, dorsal and bulbar arteries of the penis. Networks of veins drain blood into the internal iliac and pudendal veins. The autonomic and somatic nerves supply the penis.

Stimulation of the penis by the parasympathetic nerves will lead to blood engorgement and erection.

The scrotum is a superficial pouch of skin and muscles divided into two compartments, each containing a testis or male sex organ, which are responsible for the secretion of spermatozoa. During foetal development the testes descend from the abdominal cavity into the scrotum. This cooler environment is essential for normal spermatogenesis. Testes are suspended in the scrotum by the spermatic cord. Contained also in the scrotum is the epididymis, a convoluted tube some seven metres long. Maturity of spermatozoa occurs within the epididymis, whereby spermatozoa are either stored or reabsorbed. The epididymis leaves the testes to form the vas deferens. Contained within the vas deferens are the spermatic cord, testicular artery, testicular venous plexus and lymph vessels that maintain the testes via the spermatic cord.

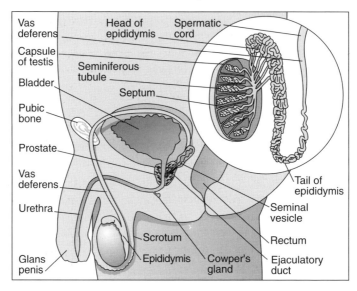

Fig 7.2 Male reproductive system

SEXUAL AROUSAL

Sexual arousal is a term widely used to describe the processes that 'turn people on', although the circumstances in which this can occur are variable. Not all forms of sexual arousal can be seen as a voluntary response to pleasure, such as physical contact by kissing. Arousal can occur while watching a film or, for example, in nursing, where a female nurse is tending to a male patient and the genitalia are exposed. An erection occurs, causing embarrassment to all concerned. How we react in such situations is important and will be referred to later in this chapter.

The term is widely used to cover a range of psychological and physiological states. Bancroft (1989) suggests an analogy to that of hunger whereby the hungry person has an appetite motivating him towards food. Within this subjective experience, the longer we are without food the more our appetite will increase. This comparison equated to sex suggests that the longer we go without it the more we will seek it. The sequence of physiological events, however, is not quite so simple. Sexual desire can be affected either negatively or positively by external stimuli, such as fantasy, odour and psychological and physical responses. Preparation for reproduction and sexual union could be seen as the goal for sexual arousal. This biological function, while important to some, is not the ultimate achievement for many. Intimacy for many couples can arouse emotions and feelings resulting in personal satisfaction and development. Masters and Johnson (1995) suggest that the process of sexual union evolves in a sequential but complex manner, which includes a series of physiological events. Changes that occur and can affect the whole body are predominately in the genital area and can be neurological, hormonal, muscular and vascular. Bancroft (1989), however, notes that the occurrence of a genital response is not always an indication of sexual arousal.

Orgasm itself is a subjective experience and the least understood. In the postpubertal male, for instance, the occurrence of ejaculation clearly marks the event. For the female there is often uncertainty whether or not an orgasm has occurred. Achievement of orgasm is culturally significant and often seen as the goal of sexual activity to conclude the experience. The inability to achieve an orgasm can therefore cause considerable anxiety to some people. Direct stimulation of the genitalia or masturbation, which are not necessarily during sexual activity, does not appear to differ physiologically (Bancroft 1989). It is also worth noting that orgasmic pleasure can have the same motivating effect in women as in men. In the female multi-orgasms are possible, whereas in the male the time between orgasm and the ability to regain an erection may be a few minutes in a healthy young male; for an elderly person it may be several hours or days.

Male arousal

Masters et al (1995) propose a four stage model which currently appears acceptable and, although physiological responses are not so separable, does assist with the identification and diagnosis of erectile problems. The four stages are:

▶ excitement

▶ plateau

▶ orgasm

▶ resolution

Currently there are still some misunderstandings on the precise mechanism of how penile erection occurs. It is known that with stimulation the arteries within the corpora cavernosa become relaxed allowing an increase in the flow of blood into the cavernosal spaces. Erection occurs when the penis becomes engorged with blood. Contraction of the muscles surrounding the penis provides further rigidity. To achieve and maintain an erection demands an intact autonomic nervous system as four coordinating processes are involved: erection, emission, ejaculation and detumescence.

Penile erection may also result from a psychological stimulus (psychogenic erection) such as erotic fantasies or visual images. This occurs via the sympathetic and parasympathetic nerves. Tactile stimulation triggers a reflexogenic response initiated by the nerves which lie in the fatty tissue within the side wall of the rectum, known as the hypogastric plexus. Emission, which is the first stage of erection, is controlled primarily by the parasympathetic nervous system. Ejaculation occurs when the seminal fluid is propelled along the urethra and expelled from the body. This is activated when closure of the bladder neck and stimulation of the parasympathetic nerve cause rhythmic contraction of the striated ischiocavernosa and bulbocavernosa muscles.

A build up of body tension, which is subsequently released, followed by a feeling of intense pleasure, can usually be referred to as orgasm. Orgasm may, however, be experienced without ejaculation or erection; it should also be noted that ejaculation could occur without the penis becoming erect. Following orgasm, ejaculation is imminent, usually within 1–3 minutes.

The phase when the genitalia return to their pre-excitory state is described as detumescence.

Female arousal

Women will undergo similar phases of physiological activity. The excitement or desire phase is indicated by vascular engorgement and swelling of the genital area, in particular the labia, in direct response to stimulation. At the same time there are muscular contractions and vasocongestion of the skin and genitalia, which can increase sensitivity to other parts of the body, including the breasts. Vaginal lubrication occurs in response to this process. The amount of vaginal lubrication is not an indicator of the level in which a woman is aroused and cannot determine that the woman is ready for male penetration of the penis. Lubrication does, however, enable the penis to be inserted more easily and without discomfort. This is then succeeded by the plateau phase where a levelling of sexual tensions will occur necessary to trigger off orgasm, a total body response with the tensions accumulated being discharged. Resolution or final phase occurs in response to this maximum level of excitement with the body returning to its former unaroused state.

EFFECTS OF MUTILATING SURGERY ON BODY IMAGE AND SEXUALITY

Patients undergoing stoma formation face permanent changes to their accepted body image, lifestyle and sexuality. Sexuality is integrally linked to the concepts of body image, self-concept, self-esteem and self-worth. Changes in physical appearance may make an individual feel less attractive. These feelings can give rise to insecurity, lack of confidence and being 'out of control'; these, in turn, can be a threat to existing relationships and friendships. Stoma surgery therefore has a profound effect on the mind as well as the body. What is seen as a physical problem will transpose into a psychological sequalae, which goes beyond the ability to engage in sexual intercourse.

What is body image?

According to Newell (1991) the concept of body image is poorly defined but does involve aspects of neurology, sociology and psychology. Several factors can affect body image and, as noted by Price (1986), include genetics, socialisation, culture, race, fashion, the media and health education. Body image can be conceptualised as a 'mental picture of one's own body, an interpersonal experience', or 'the way in which the body appears to self'; in other words what we carry in our mind (Wood, 1975). How we see and feel about ourselves – self-concept – will affect the way an individual accepts any changes to their normal body image. Schain (1980) argues that self-concept consists of four components, namely:

▶ The *body self*, which includes physical function and body image.

▶ The *interpersonal self* concerned with sexual and psychosocial interaction.

▶ The *achievement self* which considers individual status and function, such as the nature and source of employment and role in life.

▶ The *identification self* which relates to personal, ethical and spiritual beliefs.

These four areas will have an influence on a person's acceptance of body image. Every individual is unique in the way in which they see themselves, how others relate to them and how they communicate with each other. The appearance of other people can therefore influence how an individual feels and sees him or herself, and affect their perception of others. This infers that if a 'normal' person has problems with their body image, a person whose body image undergoes a change is more at risk (Salter, 1991). McCrea (1984) questioned these facts by suggesting that people with body image problems should not have to undergo such mental anxiety, and asked whether it is disease or society that causes the problems.

Concepts of body image and society norms, such as pretty and ugly, normal and different, are developed during early childhood. Throughout these formative years the attitudes of society, parents and peers will influence the way in which an adolescent regards him or herself. For example, stress may be placed on physical abilities, which will be a problem if a disability occurs in later life. Most people are self critical about their body image to some degree and, in the extreme, this can give rise to feelings of insecurity. Successful survival is dependent on the need to feel confident and be in control of their lives.

Gastrointestinal or urological illness, surgery and formation of a stoma represent a major transition in patient's lives, each stage having the potential for primary and secondary psychological problems. Wade (1990) infers that patients facing stoma surgery also face the future with a change in bodily appearance and loss of elimination control. Research to compare the psychological effects of people with continent stoma suggests that many of the body image problems related to conventional stoma have been erased, and no evidence of major problems with sexual function have been recorded (Salter, 1996).

In life it is not only necessary to adapt to changing patterns of normal body image but also to an altered body image (Price, 1990). The literature therefore suggests that there is more to an altered body image than physical effects which cannot be detached from psychological, sexual and social implications. Anxiety and depression can compound these and any other previously existing problems.

EFFECTS OF SURGERY AND/OR ADJUVANT THERAPY ON MALE SEXUAL FUNCTION

Impairment of sexual function may occur after any major stress, but this should improve in time. If there is a risk of sexual dysfunction it is the responsibility of the surgeon to discuss this with patient and partner before surgery. This allows time for the couple to discuss the possible major impact on their future lives. Ideally specialist sexual counselling should be available and the opportunity for sperm banking should be offered, supported by clear verbal and written information on access and disposal. Sexual function may be impaired prior to diagnosis, surgery or treatment; vague discomfort, pain and general malaise can contribute to a decrease in sexual desire and love making. Patients should be informed that following major surgery, with or without additional treatment, they can initially expect to experience similar feelings resulting in a potential loss of libido and sexual desire.

Erectile dysfunction (the inability to have or sustain an erection) in males may be temporary or permanent, depending on why stoma surgery is being performed. Surgery for ulcerative colitis with formation of ileostomy should not alter sexual function, whereas surgery for pelvic or bladder cancer is more extensive with possible damage to the prostatic nerve plexus; the parasympathetic and sympathetic nerves, which lie in close proximity to the bladder and rectum, are critical for erection. The autonomic nerves, which control the blood supply to the penis, can be damaged in pelvic surgery, resulting in sensory loss, a further contributor to erectile failure. Research by Joels (1989) states that sexual dysfunction occurs in 43% of male colostomy patients and virtually all following radical cystectomy for cancer.

Vascular insufficiency following radiotherapy treatment for pelvic cancer can contribute to the cause of erectile failure. Other factors to consider are the pre-existing pathology, such as diabetes, and medications that may block testosterone action, such as cimetidene for the treatment of gastric/duodenal ulcers (Leiblum and Rosen, 1992).

Total pelvic exenteration, which involves removal of all organs in the pelvic cavity, including the rectum, bladder and all male reproductive organs, results in loss of male genitalia and double stoma. Some men may not actually ejaculate whereas others experience retrograde ejaculation (dry orgasm) where the semen is ejaculated backwards into the bladder. When passing urine the colour will be changed to a 'white, milky appearance'. Men in this situation feel the intensity of orgasm but say that the experience is different.

Radiotherapy to the pelvic area can result in reduced libido, less wetness, orgasmic difficulties and infertility. Some forms of chemotherapy will have similar effects. Both will increase symptoms of lethargy, weakness and body image changes.

The psychological effects of stoma surgery can be an even greater contributor to male sexual dysfunction than the physiological and pharmacological causes. We have discussed some of the physical sequalae, which may only be apparent to the patient and their sexual partner. Chemotherapy can lead to hair loss or hormonal treatment, resulting in the development of female characteristics, such as voice changes or increased breast development. These can enhance existing effects and leave a man feeling stigmatised and distressed by fear of rejection by peers and partners. Culturally men are seen to be macho, strong and 'the breadwinner', and may feel unable to talk about their true feelings, fearful that this will be interpreted as a sign of weakness or not coping with the disease or treatment.

Table 7.1 Significant contributory factors to male sexual dysfunction

1. Loss or potential loss of sexual function is seen as a loss of manhood and the threat of not fulfilling his gender role. Men often use emotional withdrawal as a coping strategy for emotional distress.
2. Anxiety to perform and fear of rejection is a major cause of erectile failure, resulting in relationship tension and withdrawal from intimacy.
3. Depression and mood disturbance in the more debilitated patients is another cause of erectile failure.

EFFECTS OF SURGERY AND/OR ADJUVANT THERAPY ON FEMALE SEXUAL FUNCTION

The condition necessitating surgery and the type and technique of stoma surgery performed can both affect the degree of sexual/psychological problems encountered and have implications for nursing practice. A woman who has had an ileostomy for long-standing ulcerative colitis, where the chronic symptoms will have had significant impact on lifestyle activities, will probably approach surgery more positively than a woman recently diagnosed with rectal cancer requiring a colostomy. Many nurses recognise that patients are facing a life crisis but as Copey et al (1992) found in their study of gynaecological patients, nearly one-third of the women would have liked more information on the operation's effects on sexual function and indicated preference of partner involvement. Medical and health professionals generally see the effects of surgery, medication or adjuvant cancer therapy on female sexual functions as a low priority. Borwell (1996) in her study on specialist stoma care nurses found that if the issue of sexuality was raised prior to surgery, impairment to male sexual function would be acknowledged.

Women with rectal cancer who undergo abdominal perineal excision of rectum with permanent colostomy can possibly experience shortening and narrowing of the vagina. It is not surprising that when intercourse is resumed after surgery, a degree of dyspareunia (painful intercourse) will be experienced. An unhealed perineal wound or discomfort around the perineum may inhibit coitus (penetrative sex). Another possible result of this type of surgery is loss of genital sensation due to peripheral nerve damage and vaginal dryness. Dyspareunia can also occur due to anatomical changes, such as damage to the posterior vaginal wall or shortening of the vaginal vault, or decrease in the volume of vaginal secretions. Total pelvic exenteration, involving the removal of uterus, Fallopian tubes, ovaries, bladder, rectum and vagina, is considered at cancer diagnosis or recurrence when the disease is thought to be resectable and will have a profound and severe effect on function. The formation of a urinary and faecal stoma has further body image, self-esteem and sexual implications. Additional considerations are the rationale for undertaking this drastic form of surgery and the attraction of a final attempt to cure. Initially sexuality may not be perceived as a problem, with thoughts and energies being focused on survival. Research conducted by Anderson and Hacker (1983) identified a reduction in the frequency of sexual activity, low sexual arousal and satisfaction, and disruption of body image and confidence. Following total pelvic clearance women are unable to resume sexual activity if they have not undergone vaginal reconstruction.

Radiotherapy to the pelvic/vaginal area will have an effect on vaginal secretions, thinning of the vaginal lining and loss of vaginal elasticity. There is also an increased risk of vaginal fibrosis and stenosis (narrowing of the vaginal introit), resulting in dyspareunia and orgasmic difficulties. Depending on a woman's menstrual status, infertility could also be a future problem.

Chemotherapy may cause similar problems depending on the types of drugs used. General malaise, lethargy and weight loss are a realistic expectation following major surgery and, as previously stated, should be included in the pre-treatment phase information package. Surgical intervention with or without adjuvant therapy will enhance body image problems and can be a constant reminder of the underlying disease.

Nursing assessment and advice on the management of vaginal dryness should consider the pre-disposing factors to which the condition relates, for example a woman with gynaecological cancer would not usually be treated with an oestrogen based cream. There are several commercially produced water-soluble lubricants, reducing discomfort to encourage lovemaking. A disadvantage could be the anticipation that coitus will take place. An alternative spontaneous recommendation would be the use of saliva, always readily available, which can enhance lovemaking if offered by the partner. Regular use of a vaginal dilator with a water-soluble lubricant can also help to prevent vaginal stenosis. Identifying problems concerned with fear, discomfort or pain while making love will enable the nurse to discuss adopting different positions to enhance comfort. The superior position allows the woman to have greater control over the timing and degree of penetration.

Following a debilitating illness another contributor to pain and discomfort is often caused by undetected conditions such as monilial vulvovaginitis, a fungal infection (thrush). Monilia are commonly found in the vagina but may proliferate if treatment for another condition involves the use of some antibiotics, which can disturb the normal mucosal flora. Symptoms experienced are intense burning and itching of the vulval area; a thick curd-like discharge may also be present. An antifungicidal topical preparation is an effective remedy for this condition with an emphasis on personal hygiene. A typical incident recently occurred involving a seventy-year-old woman who had undergone panproctocolectomy for long-standing ulcerative colitis. While promoting and discussing aspects of care, comments were made relating to discomfort and irritation around the perineum. Examination revealed an extensive monilial infection, and yet both nurses and medical staff had reviewed the area for wound healing without comment, in spite of the patient's reference to soreness around her genitalia.

Homosexual patients

The homosexual patient with a stoma does have the same needs for information about ostomy surgery and its implications. There can be problems about disclosure of sexual orientation and sensitive concerns, making it more difficult for them to receive help. It is important to distinguish the nature of the homosexual relationship and who is the recipient in the relationship. In the patient who has had the rectum removed and is the reciprocal partner, the couple should be warned about the dangers of having penetrative sex via the stoma. Anal intercourse for some homosexuals is a source of great pleasure and possible sexual identity (Savage, 1987) but this is no longer possible following perineal excision of rectum.

INFLUENCES OF SURGERY ON BODY IMAGE AND SEXUALITY

Factors affecting both genders, whatever their sexual orientation, often relate to a feeling and fear of rejection of the stoma by their partner. Discussion of positive attributes and on how to restore confidence will help to increase self-esteem and the belief that there is life after stoma surgery. At the same time the changes which have occurred as a result of surgery or disease need to be acknowledged. Practical suggestions could include ways to enhance personal presentation and attractiveness to a partner, which will raise an individual's confidence and self-esteem. For a woman suggestions on how to achieve this could include wearing pretty lingerie, using a pouch cover or an opaque pouch to disguise the contents or introduction to a smaller style of pouch. Other tips should focus on pouch security, ensuring the pouch is emptied prior to love making, thus reducing distress and embarrassment from leakage.

Psychological factors may also predispose to a reduction or cessation in sexual activity affected by the changes to body image, diagnosis, or nonacceptance of the stoma itself. Adjustment following ostomy surgery has been investigated widely; the documented areas of concern are those that relate to sexual attractiveness. Fears have been expressed about odour, noise and appliance leakage during sexual activity (Druss et al, 1968). Other concerns relate to the reaction of a partner, fertility and childbearing (Dyk and Sutherland, 1956; Gruner et al, 1977).

Expressing sexuality is much more than intercourse alone – it is a source of human contact, comfort, and security, a measure of self-worth, providing cohesion within a relationship. The nursing diagnosis acknowledges 'altered body image' in the care plans of patients who will experience disfigurement due either to surgery or subsequent treatments, such as radiotherapy, chemotherapy or the disease process itself. This assumes that every nurse will know what constitutes a change in body image and how it is related to health. Based on these assumptions it also implies that nurses should have understanding and are equipped with the appropriate skills to offer some form of counselling (Mellor, 1996). Research on the nursing and medical profession in this area, however, would argue to the contrary that open discussion about sexuality and other areas seen to be of a sensitive nature remains uncommon. It is thought that as many as 84% of surgeons fail to invite open discussion about potential sexual difficulties before surgery (Rubin and Devlin, 1987). These issues are rarely raised by nurses, family doctors or junior hospital doctors, so patients often discover their physical malfunction postoperatively and suffer additional psychological trauma. This reluctance by health professionals to discuss sexual issues is further recognised by Webb (1985a) and Borwell (1996), and as Woods (1975) infers, 'loss of control of a bodily function such as that experienced by ostomates generates anxiety about adult sex role identification and social interaction'.

The bereavement process is a common analogy used to describe the feelings and emotions that these patients and their families will undergo (Kubler-Ross, 1970; Bowlby, 1980; Buckman, 1992). Gloeckner (1984) identified that over half of the respondents to his research noted a decrease in feelings of sexual attractiveness and unacceptability in the first year after surgery. The implications for nurses and health professionals in the management of ostomy patients are therefore evident.

REHABILITATION AND THERAPEUTIC HELPING IN NURSING

Ill health is associated with impaired sexuality. However it is also apparent that a decline in sexual health is not dependent on poor health. Equally, good health does not depend on sexuality as often supposed – many people are sexually inactive and will vary according to individual, personal characteristics.

Stoma patients have the potential to experience clinically significant psychological problems following surgery, which frequently are not recognised by health professionals, such as surgeons and stoma care nurses. Preoperative preparation and continuity of care following discharge, particularly for those with an increased risk of psychiatric morbidity, is critical if these current statistics are to be improved (White and Hunt, 1997; Wade, 1989). Psychological disturbance to sexual function is mainly rooted in feelings of guilt, fear, anger, anxiety and depression. Lack of knowledge, embarrassment and ineffective communication by the nurse can contribute to these difficulties.

Any anxieties that the patient, their partner or children may have will need to be explored. These could be related to their feelings about lifestyle activities, employment, personal relationships and possible changes that the future may bring. Some couples do have difficulty in communicating with each other about sexual anxieties. Many patients admit being aware of stigma to a degree (Devlin et al, 1971; Macdonald, 1982); they no longer see themselves as 'normal', resulting in withdrawal from social contact.

Rehabilitation requires the nurse to have knowledge of or access to current information about when to resume sexual activity, and resources and aids available for male and female sexual dysfunction.

Following major pelvic surgery it is usually agreed that sexual activity can safely be resumed once healing of the perineum has occurred. This is usually determined at the post-discharge follow-up clinic, approximately six weeks postoperatively. Physical weakness is commonly experienced by patients in this phase; being sexually active is not always seen as a priority. Performance anxiety and fear of failure between a couple can be associated with sexual difficulties and not physical impairment. Information should also reinforce the need for a realistic time span for nerves and other structures to recover before any permanent estimation of dysfunction can be determined. Preoperative assessment should have identified any existing sexual problems relating to pharmacology or other conditions that can be dealt with in an appropriate manner.

In the male with erectile dysfunction, intracavernosal injection therapy and vacuum and constriction devices have been available for some time with varying degrees of success. Couples who are motivated, prepared to practise and receptive to changes in their sexual activity to include the device are most likely to achieve success. Penile prostheses can be a positive means of providing an erection following disease or injury, offering a more natural solution to erectile dysfunction, but they do have their limitations. Pharmacology and the new oral agents are the current shift for the treatment of erectile disorders. Sildenafil (Viagra) has received a controversial reception in the United Kingdom, largely due to the financial implications and lack of guidance on its administration. Sildenafil is effective in treating erectile dysfunction of broad aetiology but does require a thorough patient assessment prior to usage.

Successful pregnancies are possible depending on the type of surgical technique. Contraception and preconceptual advice should be addressed when assessing premenopausal women. Intrauterine devices are not usually recommended, oral contraception being preferable, although absorption may be affected. This can be determined by the type of operation or the particular contraceptive pill prescribed.

There is minimal evidence regarding the pharmacological advantages in the treatment of female sexual dysfunction. Sildenafil and other oral agents have been proposed as beneficial agents due to their enhancing effect on vasocongestion of the vagina and clitoris.

LEARNING TO ASK

Nurses generally will inform their (male) patients of the potential physical effects of ostomy surgery on sexual function, irrespective of the fact that this problem may already have been in existence for some time. Assessment can legitimise the patient's sexual concerns, and clarify and reinforce diagnosis, terminology, prognosis and proposed treatment, including any side effects.

The following considerations are relevant for the stoma patient:

▶ past and current physical status;

▶ patient's psychosocial and sexual status;

▶ their current psychological status;

▶ their current social status.

Within these factors are the attitude of the partner toward the stoma and their emotional and physical health which are all intertwined (Coates, 1989). Lomont et al (1978) also acknowledged the importance of an educated and informed partner in total sexual rehabilitation. Where appropriate it is important to include the partner in teaching sessions. Commonly, focus is on a patient's sexuality and the potential effects of the partner are frequently overlooked. The 'well' partner can also suffer from fatigue, be hesitant to initiate a relationship for fear of causing pain or damage to the 'ill' partner and may feel guilty. Within sexual counselling (or helping) in nursing the main objective is to provide an insight into an individual's pattern of communication and interaction. As patients progress through the rehabilitation period, non-intrusive questioning in follow-up can establish how well they are reintegrating back into their previous lifestyle. Observation on a person's appearance, voice and mood can help nurses assess how well they are managing. Assessing the extent of their sexual difficulty can sometimes be a problem as there can be a reluctance to talk about intimate problems, hence the importance of a sexual health assessment as part of the overall care. A nurse who feels comfortable while listening, and who encourages and shares her knowledge, can help to clarify sexual problems, consider solutions or maybe compromise and give permission for the patient to consider changes in established patterns of sexual expression.

Adaptation of a recognised framework such as the PLISSIT model (Annon, 1974) can offer an assessment tool to be used with patients and will also provide a way in which nurses can identify their own strengths and weaknesses to action other more appropriate agencies.

Table 7.2 PLISSIT Framework

P. –	Permission (giving)	EXPLORATION
L. I. –	Limited Information	UNDERSTANDING
S. S. –	Specific Suggestions	ACTION
I. T. –	Intensive Therapy	

Permission (the beginning, exploratory stage)

Patients with sexual difficulties or issues to be discussed relating to their medical condition may need permission to: acknowledge they need help; discuss sex; feel that they are respected for who they are and can raise issues which concern their sexual behaviour and relationships; have complex feelings.

Permission giving requires the nurse to be:

▶ sensitive and use the skills of active listening;

▶ introduce and initiate discussion by adopting a direct and explicit approach, using language that the patient understands, modelling her knowledge of sexual language and behaviour.

Offering patients the freedom to talk about their sexual concerns will help them to clarify what the actual and potential problems are and will form the basis of assessment for any future counselling or support.

Limited Information (in the understanding stage)

Information already acquired will enable the nurse to assess what difficulties are being experienced, whether to engage in further discussion or counselling or if patients should be referred for more expert help. Sexual counselling explores the deeper insights, awareness and understanding of the patient's problem. A patient may, for example, disclose that he is homosexual and will want to know how having a colostomy will affect his relationships with other homosexuals. At this stage the nurse will probably need to supply additional, relevant information which could be written details of appropriate associations, such as SPOD (Sexual and Personal problems Of the Disabled). This type of information cannot compensate for the interaction between patient and nurse, but it will support and provide another dimension. Offered with sensitivity this type of information can often liberate patients and provide the freedom to express their sexual concerns and difficulties. At the end of this intervention patients should be able to recognise their sexual behaviour as an expression of the dynamics of a relationship and, where appropriate, be offered an opportunity to communicate this to their partner. Giving limited information is an important part of the sexual counselling process and can contribute to the insights and patterns of communication and interaction.

Specific Suggestions (in the action stage)

Some patients will need more than permission and information. For example, the patient who has disclosed his homosexuality and has undergone excision of rectum with a permanent colostomy will possibly need assistance with understanding new practices of sexual behaviour. This should take the form of involving the other partner in a relationship to help with negotiated tasks designed to enhance communication between the couple. A necessary requisite for the resolution of sexual problems is the creation of a humanised sexual system (Kaplan, 1974). The essential ingredients are open communication and the expression of feelings that portray a genuine willingness between the couple for correcting and resolving such problems. Developing these abilities will help patients respond more effectively to their sexual concerns.

Intensive Therapy (a behavioural based action stage)

Nearly every patient will benefit from counselling with a sexual focus, through which permission is given and the information acquired is used to enhance further understanding and gain deeper insights into the patient's particular sexual problems. There is a group of patients who will require specific systematic behavioural programmes designed to change sexual behaviour and function. This group needs the skills of a recognised sex therapist that can offer intensive therapy tailored to their individual needs. Nurses and other health professionals who have identified and acknowledged this need with their patients are responsible for ensuring a smooth transition to an appropriately qualified therapist. (Adaptation of RELATE handout, 1993, Annon, 1974)

SEXUAL HEALTH ASSESSMENT IN COMMUNITY CARE

Assessment should include a description of past patterns of sexual expression, recent changes in activity, knowledge of illness, related changes in sexual function and beliefs about sexual expression. An individual's concern about sexuality will not necessarily be associated with a change in sexual function. It is, however, necessary to determine an individual's and their partner's degree of satisfaction or dissatisfaction in fulfilling their sexual needs.

Many authors suggest a full history should be taken from everyone. Various restraints play an integral part of physical/psychosocial functioning, in particular, time, embarrassment on the part of nurse/patient and lack of general acceptance of sexuality.

▶ *Timing* is important in the acceptance by the patient when raising issues that have a sensitive connotation. It has been noted that the optimal time is not on initial interaction with the patient but it could be argued that a sexual history should be taken alongside a nursing/medical history. The following suggestions could form a useful criterion:

▶ *Age* – considerations should include the very young and elderly widows/widowers, as it may be inappropriate within some of these groups. However it is mandatory for those in late adolescence and people in an existing relationship. Individuals not in a current relationship should not be excluded on these factors alone: thinking about future relationships when presenting with an illness or other medical condition can be an added source of anxiety.

▶ *Gender* – there may be differences in how this is approached between men and women when undertaking assessment.

▶ *Context* of consultation will influence who is interviewed, and the reason for and timing of presentation.

▶ *Conservatism* – this can be the greatest barrier on the part of patient/practitioner. Again nurses should exercise the skill of being non-judgemental about their patients.

Where to take a sexual health assessment

Within the clinical setting this can create many barriers, for example lack of privacy, noise, interruptions and the sensitivity of the issue. In community practice there will be other considerations relating to the environment, timing and privacy. Confidentiality should be assured at all times and choosing the appropriate 'moment', that is not when a patient already feels threatened or vulnerable.

Language

Do not invite a negative response by asking questions such as, 'Have you ever...?'Patients will also not expect nurses to use 'slang' words. Check out the patients understanding of terminology before you start. 'Sleeping with someone' may mean having penetrative sex or it could mean being close in a relationship and just sleeping in the same bed. When referring to parts of the sexual anatomy, drawings can be a useful way of illustrating anatomical parts. Homosexual behaviour has been commonly thought to mean anal intercourse. Use open questions to elicit a response, for example: 'Is there anything else at all you would like to ask or tell me about? If you should think of anything later, do mention it to me or anyone else you feel can help.'

Once you are in discussion, additional questions can be used for each problem mentioned: 'Could you tell me a little more about that?' 'When did that first happen?' 'How do you think people can help you with...?' (Adapted from Webb, 1985)

Teamwork

The concept of working together in healthcare indicates important messages for planners, managers and practitioners. Interprofessional work raises many issues. Carrier and Kendall (1995) identify a tension in conceptualising multiprofessional work as a cooperative enterprise in which traditional forms and divisions of professional knowledge and authority are retained. A more radical review of interprofessional work implies a willingness to share and give up exclusive claims to specialised knowledge and authority if other professional groups can meet the needs of clients more efficiently. Focusing on the ostomy patient, health policy demonstrates a shift from disease management and an illness service to emphasis on health and its promotion. Each major professional group proclaims that health promotion lies at the foundation of their work and is an important part of their roles.

CONCLUSION

The aim of the nurse as a therapeutic helper is to improve patient care. According to Corner (1997) the features most common to this development are:

▶ Adopts an integrated view of the individual.

▶ Offers care that is participative, collaborative and empowering.

▶ Undertakes deconstruction of the environment/system of care to enable radical changes in caring to take place.

▶ Involves reflection and evaluation of the process of nursing.

▶ Focus of care should be need/problem oriented.

▶ Aims to move individuals towards healing and health in the broadest sense.

One of the most important improvements in care might be more sensitive and thoughtful attention to the frequency and quality of communication with the patient.

Once discharged appointments will be made for surveillance by medical staff and the specialist stoma care nurse within a specified time frame. If the patient does not attend, this will be documented and investigated. Many stoma care nurses manage direct access referrals and clinics for patients who have physically related stoma problems or other concerns.

There are always many causative factors present; sometimes these can be attached to the current situation, for example long term relationship disharmony. What needs to be defined for a management programme is a thorough exploration of a couple's attitudes and values to identify the root cause of sexual dysfunction. One must also consider other predisposing and precipitating factors such as the patient/partner who does not want to resume sexual functioning.

Example: A woman in her early fifties had an active sex life with her husband and through discussion it was explained that there should be no reason why this would change after surgery. Her comment: 'Please don't tell my husband that. Having this operation can be an excuse not to have sex any more.'

Management of sexual problems following stoma surgery has to acknowledge that any physical effects of sexual dysfunction will be psychologically interrelated and are inseparable.

Learning outcomes

▶ The impact of stoma surgery and treatment on sexuality.

▶ The problems that may arise following stoma surgery on a person's sexuality.

▶ Why patients undergoing stoma surgery incur changes in sexual function.

▶ Strategies that can have a positive influence on patient care.

▶ The nurse's role in promoting a healthy sexuality.

'How well the patient functions sexually after we have finished with him will depend largely on how effective we have been. If sexuality is part of the quality of life, then healthcare professionals can no longer ignore these components of nursing care.' (Wells, 1990)

REFERENCES

Anderson, B.L., Hacker, N. (1983) Psychosexual adjustment following pelvic exenteration. *Journal of Obstetrics and Gynaecology;* 61: 3, 331–338.

Annon, J.S. (1974) *The Behavioural Treatment of Sexual Problems.* Vol.1, Brief Therapy. Honolulu: Enabling Systems.

Bancroft, J. (1989) *Human Sexuality and its Problems.* London: Churchill Livingstone.

Borwell, B. (1996) *The provision of counselling and sexual health.* (Masters Dissertation) University of Southampton.

Bowlby, J. (1980) *Attachment and Loss: Sadness and Depression.* Vol.111, New York, N.Y.: Basic Books.

Buckman, R. (1992) *How to Break Bad News: A Guide for Healthcare Professionals.* Basingstoke: Papermac

Coates, R. (1989) Stoma, sexuality, the patient and the practitioner. *Journal of World Council of Enterostomal Therapists;* November, 23–25.

Carrier, J. Kendall, I. (1995) Professionalism and interprofessionalism in health and community care: some theoretical issues. In: Owens, P., Carrier, J. (eds.) *Interprofessional Issues in Community and Primary Health Care.* London: Macmillan.

Copey, R., Everett, N., Howells, A. et al (1992) The care of patients undergoing surgery for gynaecological cancer. *Journal of Advanced Nursing;* 17, 667–671.

Corner, J. (1997) Beyond survival rates and side effects: cancer nursing as therapy. *Cancer Nursing;* 20: 1, 3–11.

Devlin, H.B., Plant, J.A., Griffen, M. (1971) Aftermath of surgery for rectal cancer. *British Medical Journal;* iii, 413–418.

Druss, R., O'Connor, J., Prudden, J. et al (1968) *Archives of General Psychiatry;* 18, 53–59.

Dyk, R., Sutherland, A. (1956) Adaptation of the spouse and other family to the colostomy patient. *Cancer;* 9, 123–138.

Elcoat, C. (1986) *Stoma Care Nursing: Current Nursing Practice.* London: Bailière Tindall.

Glen, S. (1986) Altered body image in children. In: Salter, M. (ed.) *Altered Body Image: The Nurse's Role.* 1st Edition. Chichester: John Wiley & Sons.

Gloeckner, M. (1983) Partner reaction following ostomy surgery. *Journal of Sex and Marital Therapy;* 9, 182–190.

Gregory, P. (1997) Anatomy and physiology of male/female reproductive system. In: Borwell, B. (ed.) *Developing Sexual Helping Skills.* Maidenhead, Berks.: Medical Projects International.

Joels, J. (1989) Psychosexual implications of having a stoma. *Surgical Nurse* (special supplement on stoma care); 2: 6, x–xii.

Kaplan, H.S. (1974) *The New Sex Therapy.* New York: Brunel/Mazel inc.

Kubler-Ross, E. (1970) *On Death and Dying.* London: Tavistock.

Leiblum, S.R., Rosen, R.C. (1989) *Sexual Desire Disorders.* New York: The Guilford Press.

Lomont, H.A., De Petrillo, A.D., Sargent, E.J. (1978) Psychosexual rehabilitation and extensive surgery. *Gynaecological Oncology;* 6, 236–242.

Masters, W.H., Johnson, V.E., Kolodny, R.C. (1995) *Human Sexuality.* 5th Edition. New York: Harper Collins inc.

Mellor, D. (1996) Altered Body Image. *Professional Nurse;* 11: 5, 297–298.

Moore, G.J. (1997) *Women and Cancer.* London: Jones and Bartlett International.

Newell, R. (1991) Body image disturbance: cognitive behavioural formulation and intervention. *Journal of Advanced Nursing;* 16, 1400–1405.

Price, B. (1986) *Body Image: Nursing Concepts and Care.* Hemel Hempstead: Prentice Hall.

RELATE (1993) *Handout on PLISSIT Framework.* Rugby: Relate.

Rubin, G.P., Devlin, H.B. (1987) The quality of life with a stoma. *British Journal of Hospital Medicine;* 38: 4, 300–306.

Salter, M. (1996) Sexuality and the stoma patient. In: Myers, C. (ed.) *Stoma Care Nursing: A Patient Centred Approach.* London: Edward Arnold.

Salter, M. (1991) Coming to terms with a change in body image. *Journal of W.C.E.T. Worldwide;* 2: 3, July/Sept. 16–19.

Savage, J. (1987) *Nurses, Gender and Sexuality.* London: Heinemann Nursing.

Wade, B. (1989) *A Stoma is for Life.* London: Scutari.

Wade, B. (1990) Colostomy patients' psychological adjustment at 10 weeks and 1 year after surgery in districts which employed stoma care nurses and districts which did not. *Journal of Advanced Nursing;* 15, 1297–1304.

Webb, C. (1985) *Sexuality, Nursing and Health.* Chichester: John Wiley & Sons.

Webb, C. (1985) Guidelines for taking a sexual history. In: Webb, C. *Sexuality, Nursing and Health. Chichester* : John Wiley & Sons.

Wells, R. (1990) Sexuality: an unknown word for patients with a stoma. In: Senn, H., Glens, J. (eds.) *Results in Cancer Research.* Berlin: Springer–Verlag.

White, C.A., Hunt, J.C. (1997) Psychological factors in postoperative adjustment to stoma surgery. *Annals of the Royal College of Surgeons of England;* 79, 3–7.

Woods, N. (1975) *Human Sexuality in Health and Illness.* St. Louis, MO: CV Mosby & Co.

World Health Organisation (1975) *Education and treatment in human sexuality: the training of health professionals.* (Technical Report no. 572) Geneva: WHO.

8 The role of self-help/support groups

Alan Mortiboys

ORIGINS

There are three groups for ostomists in the UK and Ireland – the British Colostomy Association (BCA), the Ileostomy and Internal Pouch Support Group (*ia*) and the Urostomy Association (UA).

The first of these to form was the *ia* at a meeting in the Board Room of the General Hospital in Birmingham on 14 April 1956. The full story of its origins is documented in fascinating detail in the booklet, 'The Rising of the Phoenix', and it is an early example of excellent cooperation between the professional, in this case the surgeon Bryan Brooke, and the patient, Doreen Harris, an ileostomist since 1947. The actual correspondence which led to the first meeting of the 'Ileostomy Club', as it was provisionally named, is presented in this booklet and confirms the vision and commitment of these two principals. The flood of tributes on Bryan Brooke's death in September 1998 emphasised his surgical innovation in revolutionising the surgical treatment of ulcerative colitis by the introduction of the Brooke ileostomy. However, they also stressed his innovation in supporting the formation of a self-help group. It was his 'firm belief, not commonly shared at the time, that patients could effectively help each other and that professionals could learn much from them in this new field of patient care' wrote one tributary (Alexander, 1998).

In 1964 the national association expanded its title to include Ireland. In 1993 in recognition of the growing numbers who had undergone the newer pouch surgery instead of an ileostomy, the title was changed to Ileostomy and Internal Pouch Support Group.

What is now BCA began in 1963 as the Colostomy Welfare Group. Again a professional was directly involved in setting up the group. Frances Goodall CBE RSN, General Secretary and subsequently Vice President of the Royal College of Nursing, formed a group of colostomists, former patients at the Royal Marsden Hospital in London, who were willing to visit new patients before their operation and to be available to assist them afterwards. This group, which Goodall organised and trained, became in demand at other hospitals in London and then beyond. It became a charity in 1967 and in 1989 the group changed its name and constitution to become the British Colostomy Association.

The idea for UA seems to have begun at an *ia* meeting in Manchester in May 1971. Once again, a collaboration between a patient, Valerie Kings, and a professional, Laurie Kenefick – then a charge nurse at the hospital – was the basis for the formation of the association. Their conversation at the *ia* meeting led to the first meeting of the Urinary Conduit Association at The Christie Hospital and Holt Radium Institute in September 1971. Until then urostomates could be associate members of *ia*, or might belong to the CWG, but had no groups of their own. The first president, Mr Raymond Carroll, describes UA as a 'sister organisation' to *ia*. It changed its name to the Urostomy Association in 1985.

All three associations are registered charities and are themselves members of the International Ostomy Association (IOA). IOA, which describes itself as an association for ostomy associations, came into being in 1976.

In early 1999 BCA had a membership of 14,000, *ia* 10,000 and UA a steady membership of 2,500.

A related organisation, operating on a smaller scale than the three above, is the National Advisory Service for Parents of Children with a Stoma (NASPCS). In existence in one form or another since 1984, and a registered charity since 1988, the organisation has over 600 family members. It provides information via leaflets and booklets, primarily on the birth conditions that can necessitate stomas for children, as well as a newsletter and contact list for members. It is a wholly voluntary association without membership fees or any other form of funding.

STRUCTURE AND FUNDING

ia and UA are very similar in structure, reflecting the origins of UA from within *ia*. Each nationally has a medical president as do all of their branches (UA) or divisions (ia). Committees from each local group send a delegate to the National Annual General Meeting (NAGM) for UA or National Council for *ia*. This meeting votes for the Executive Committee. The Executive Committee's functions are to run the association's day-to-day affairs, and to generate ideas and recommend matters of policy to the membership, usually via the national meetings, for the further development of the association. Responsibilities of the members of the Executive Committees cover a number of specific functions or areas of concern, some of which have national sub-committees. The UA's National Executive Committee's posts comprise President, Chairman, Secretary, Treasurer, Journal Editor, Fund Raising Officer, Stoma Care Liaison Officer, Young Persons' Advisor and elected member's representatives. *ia*'s National Committee has posts identical in name and/or function to these, and in addition a Publicity Coordinator, Finance Sub-committee Chairman, Visiting Coordinator, Ostomy Care Products Secretary, Welfare Officer, International Relations Secretary, Exhibitions Coordinator and Pouch Groups Representative.

In both associations the National Secretary is a full-time salaried post. In *ia* the post is funded from within the association; while the UA National Secretary's post is funded by Macmillan Cancer Relief via BCA. *ia* also employs a National Treasurer who is almost full time. Both UA and *ia* charge a small annual subscription to members.

UA has 29 local branches. The local groups of *ia*, currently numbering 58, moved from branch to division status in 1993, influenced by changes in laws relating to charities.

BCA does not charge subscriptions to members; it first received funding from the National Society for Cancer Relief, now Macmillan Cancer Relief, in 1974. A central team of four full-time paid workers comprises a Director of Operations, a National Services Coordinator, a Treasurer and an Association Secretary. This team coordinates the work of the volunteers who make up the 26 Area Organisers, who each in turn coordinate activities of a local team of volunteers.

ACTIVITIES

All three UK associations exist to provide support for prospective, new and existing ostomists, although there are of course differences in wording and indeed emphasis within each association's aims.

BCA 'represents the interests of people with a colostomy and provides support, reassurance and practical information to anyone who is about to have a colostomy, or who already has a colostomy'.

The stated aims of UA are:

- to assist those who are about to undergo or who have undergone surgery which results in the formation of a urinary stoma;

- to assist carers in the rehabilitation of the ostomate;

- to improve the quality of life of urostomates;

- to undertake such research as the membership feels is necessary to enhance the life of urostomates.

ia describes itself as a mutual aid association with the primary aim of helping people who have had their colon removed to return to a full active and normal life as soon as possible.

With all three, it is useful to distinguish between the work carried out nationally and by local groups. Most members experience their association through local groups. They provide the opportunity to meet with others in the locality who have undergone a similar experience. For *ia* and UA, variations in the activities of each local group are most likely to depend on the individuals involved, the geographical region they cover, the size of membership and the amount of funds available. Generally there will be meetings at evenings or weekends which may have as their focus a talk, often on a relevant medical topic, and which at the same time serve as informal social gatherings. Fund-raising also takes place at a local level. Local meetings can reinforce the feeling that individual members are not unique; it is here that they can 'look to others for validation of their own feelings and attitudes' (Simpson, 1996) as well as exchanging concrete suggestions, based on personal experience, for dealing with problems. The meetings are not necessarily structured with the encouragement of these individual exchanges as a primary aim, but accommodate them happening informally and almost incidentally. Of course the meetings are most potent as a form of support for new ostomists, and a well-run event will make sure that new members are identified and fully welcomed.

These meetings also provide the opportunity for 'helper therapy' (Simpson, 1996) – the idea that by being a useful resource to another, for example an 'old' ostomist providing advice and reassurance to a 'new' ostomist, the helper can feel better about themselves and more adjusted to their situation.

BCA's local structure revolves around its Area Organisers who organise local meetings and represent the association to healthcare professionals and other interested parties. This involves them in a great deal of promotional work. Also, whenever possible they help to improve the income of Macmillan Cancer Relief. BCA does not itself run local self-help groups but facilitates their development where there is a request.

Perhaps the most important activity from the perspective of new and prospective ostomists is the role the associations perform in visiting. This activity is central to the work of all three. At any meeting of ostomists there will be several present who will recount similar tales of being visited shortly before or after surgery by an existing ostomist – they are likely to recall feelings such as relief, reassurance, encouragement or hope at seeing someone who looks 'normal'. The new ostomist is able to ask 'What's it like?' and get a response based on personal experience, which no amount of excellent information leaflets, videos and professionals can convey. The usual process that results in a visit is when a stoma care nurse makes a request for a visit from the appropriate local ostomy group. Good relationships between the stoma care nurse and the ostomy group are of course a prerequisite for the request to be made and when this does happen it is an excellent example of professionals and volunteers working together to provide a complementary service. However, given the visitor's potential to wield great influence over the patient, the role entails a high degree of responsibility. This in turn has implications for the selection and preparation of visitors – a topic returned to below.

At a national level the range of activities for all three associations is reflected in the titles of the Executive Committee posts for *ia* and UA listed above. Alongside services provided direct to and on behalf of members, both UA and *ia* fund research, usually into the illnesses which have resulted in surgery for members. *ia*'s Romania project, initiated in 1996, was an instance of international collaboration. Recognising the desperate need in Romania for the provision and services which ileostomists here often take for granted, the association set out to raise money for the express purpose of assisting development in Romania.

All three associations provide information for members, relatives, the medical profession and other interested parties. Both *ia* and UA have a journal, which appears respectively four and three times a year, while BCA produces the magazine 'Tidings' twice a year. These include news for local groups, news on developments in appliances, items of general interest and members' letters. In addition, each association provides a range of leaflets and pamphlets such as BCA's 'Living with a Colostomy', *ia*'s 'Going Home' or UA's 'Common Urostomy Problems in Pregnancy'.

It is at a national level that the associations are more likely to engage in advocacy on behalf of their members. This can take the form of representing individual members, for instance if they have experienced discrimination by employers; it may be feedback to manufacturers on behalf of users of their equipment; or it may be on behalf of the membership as a whole. Two examples of this can be found in the annual report by Tom Keily, Chairman of *ia*, in March 1999. He refers to the 'short but effective campaign' mounted with regard to prescription exemptions, which resulted in a statement from the health minister that all current prescription charge exemptions will remain in place for the life of the parliament. He goes on to cite the effective involvement of all three associations in the NHS Executive review of appliance contractor remuneration: 'The voluntary associations have made it clear that whatever the outcome of the remuneration review patients must not be asked to accept a lowering of the quality of service, standards, or a lessening of choice.' This is not a new role for the associations; they were all influential when lobbying the DHSS to create stoma care nurses, or stomatherapists as they were known when they were introduced in 1974.

IOA's activities directly reflect its aims. They are:

- to provide information and management guidelines to its Member Associations;

- to help to form new ostomy associations;

- to represent worldwide the interests of all ostomates and those with related surgeries by advocating on all ostomy-related matters and policies.

Borkman (1997) has noted the rapid changes in the self-help scene following the developments in electronic communication. A striking example of this can be found by visiting the IOA's web page at *www.ostomyinternational.org* and going into the Guest Book or Global Discussion Forum. Just as with 'real' exchanges, this provides a source of rich and useful information for the ostomist as well as that sense of not being alone. At the same time, it enables the 'outsider' to be privy to self-help and support exchanges in action. Anyone with doubts about the potential positive outcomes of such exchanges need only observe the immediate impact that direct, sensitive communication from a fellow ostomist can have in terms of reassurance, or read some of the supportive responses to requests for information or note the statements of reassurance from enquirers. It is impossible not to be moved by the urgency of some requests or by the expressions of relief or gratitude when responses are received. Borkman (1997) points out that these networks can be useful for those for whom face-to-face meetings are not possible; in addition, the partial anonymity of the participants makes it easier for those who might be reticent in 'real' social gatherings. The form is also so immediate – a request for advice or information can receive several responses from around the world within hours. If the explosion in access to and use of these forms of communication continues, some interesting questions for associations such as these ostomy groups will be raised. Will the need for local gatherings decline? Indeed will there still be a need for an ostomist to be a member of an association in order to access a network of fellow ostomists?

THE ROLE AND FUNCTION OF THE ASSOCIATIONS

Attempts to categorise these associations as self-help groups, support groups or advocacy groups can be frustrating and possibly not fruitful.

First, this is because there are no universally agreed definitions of either self-help or support groups, as noted by Bottomley (1997), 'a precise definition of a support group is not agreed', and Hildingh et al (1995), 'consensus about the meaning of the concept of social support has not been reached'.

Second, there is to some extent a distinction to be made between the associations' activities at a local and national level. The kinds of local members' meetings described above match a range of definitions of self-help and support groups. For example:

'Voluntary small group structures for mutual aid, and the accomplishment of a special purpose.' – Katz and Bender's definition of self-help groups as cited by Simpson (1996).

'A self-help group is a group of individuals who experience a common problem, share their personal stories and knowledge to help one another cope with their situation and simultaneously help and are helped.' (Gidron and Hasenfeld, 1994)

'Self-help groups are defined here as collectives of voluntarily associating persons who share a common problem; they are self-governing, rely on the experiential knowledge of their members as the group's source of authority, provide mutual assistance which is at least emotional support and do not charge fees... Voluntary mutual assistance of experiential peers with health or social issues is the essence.' (Borkman, 1997)

'Social support is an exchange between people of thoughts and services, such as instrumental aid, emotion, information and appraisal.' (Hildingh et al, 1995)

Similarly these local meetings reflect Bottomley's observation (1997) that participation in a support group produces 'mutual aid that can help the patients by providing emotional and social support, offering direct assistance, providing advice based on experiences and importantly, by providing a sense of belonging to a group'.

It should be repeated that while exchanges and mutual aid as described in these definitions can result from local gatherings, they do not necessarily happen in a structured way and they may not be the expressed purpose of the event.

At a national level, the work includes: the support of local groups; co-ordinating activities; administration of funds; support of research; provision of information and training, liaison with other groups, nationally and internationally and with the media and suppliers and manufacturers; running a helpline. The nature of these activities does not equate with a small self-help group offering emotional support and direct interaction between members. Indeed as noted above, this is the level at which some form of advocacy can be seen. While the associations' activities are not confined to a definition of an advocacy group such as 'the members' goal is to change others or the system' (Rootes and Aanes, 1992), it is clearly seen as part of their role, as indicated by the examples cited above.

Internationally, advocacy is one of the explicit concerns of IOA. This is evidenced by, for instance, IOA's support of ISCAP, the International Stoma Care Advocacy Programme. This initiative, funded by an unconditional grant from Convatec, recognises that 'stomas raise issues that go beyond the purely clinical'. It exists to 'encourage the formation, in certain countries, of working partnerships between ostomy associations, policy makers and opinion formers to encourage a greater understanding about stomas, to address aspects of policy and practice and to ensure that policy makers and opinion formers have access to accurate and relevant information about the needs of people with stomas'.

In attempting to clarify the role of these groups, we should recognise that they may not lend themselves to being understood solely in terms of self-help or support or advocacy, but to a combination of these which to some extent depends on the context in which the group is operating.

Borkman (1997) suggests three important ways in which self-help groups differ. The first of these is the extent to which they develop an alternative organisational structure to the conventional bureaucracy; clearly this has not been an issue for ostomy groups. Second, there is the extent to which their goals are primarily 'therapeutic' to support members or also include advocacy goals. As we have seen, there is an emphasis on the former, certainly at the local level, but advocacy activities are more prominent nationally. Third, there is the extent to which they cooperate with professionals and with mainstream services and it is this crucial aspect of the associations' work that is now addressed.

RELATIONSHIPS WITH PROFESSIONALS

A spectrum of attitudes towards professionals by self-help groups has been noted, for example by Borkman (1997): 'Some challenge professional ideology and practices whereas others uncritically complement professional services.' Clearly the associations under discussion here are not of the former type. They still approximate to the US ostomy groups described in 1970 as 'a community resource, working in collaboration with hospital professionals, as an adjunct to existing resources' (Lenneberg and Rowbotham, cited in Simpson, 1996).

Generally the associations make use of the kind of aid that professionals can offer. Examples listed by Yoak and Chesler include: 'helping groups to be formed, lending support and consultation, training members for leadership roles, and giving ongoing service' (Hildingh et al, 1995). It seems that the majority of ostomy association members and professionals involved in ostomy surgery and ostomy care recognise the benefits in complementing each other. This is a far cry from the days when the associations began. Nancy Alexander recalls criticisms made of Bryan Brooke in the 1950s when he supported the development of *ia*, as such groups were thought of as 'subversive, anti-authoritarian, given to hypochondria' (Alexander, 1998).

However, barriers can exist which Simpson (1996) notes stem from 'lack of knowledge, interaction and understanding'. She advises that where they do exist these barriers should be understood by both parties.

Perhaps the most basic potential barrier is that professionals don't know about the association(s) – 'the biggest problem with professionals is they do not know they have something to learn about self-help groups.' (Borkman, 1997) The same author comments earlier on professionals' ignorance of the differences between member-run self-help groups and professionally run support groups. It is for the associations to take the initiative here. They have recognised this as evidenced by, for example, BCA's Area Organisers taking a prominent role in promoting the work of the organisation or *ia* having a Publicity Coordinator post in its Executive Committee.

A second and more likely barrier is that professionals know of the association(s) but don't value them. Simpson (1996) outlines Borkman's notions of professional truth versus experiential truth. Professional truth is: 'the knowledge developed, applied and transmitted by an established, specialised occupation. Access to this knowledge is limited to those who have met the requirements of specialised education and training in a discipline, and who possess the appropriate credentials.' Experiential truth is knowledge 'based on an individual's actual experience... more or less representative of the experience of others who have the same problem' – in this case, having the illness, undergoing surgery and most importantly living with a stoma. It can be difficult for an individual whose training and, indeed, own status emphasise professional truth to acknowledge the value of another truth beyond theirs. 'Professionals need to know about... the role of experiential knowledge, and its value to patients regaining and maintaining health status' (Simpson, 1996). If the stance of some self-help groups can be seen as anti-professional, the potential for professionals to be anti-experiential must be recognised too. If this barrier is to be overcome, it might be best dealt with in the professionals' training programmes. Hildingh et al (1995) note the potential problem of lack of preparation of professionals for the appropriate roles for them in relation to self-help groups. Simpson (1996) endorses this by suggesting that 'education and training on consumer issues should be established within all professional courses in order that each individual may acquire a balanced view'. This could include more exposure of the professionals in their training to those with experiential knowledge.

A further barrier to cooperation may be when the professionals know of the groups and value them but, perhaps quite reasonably, have anxieties about exposing patients to well-intentioned volunteers who have valuable experiential knowledge but do not necessarily know how best to use it. For this reason, training given by associations to members likely to be involved in helping is of vital importance. In light of the potential influence of the visitor noted above, it is perhaps in this area that training is most important. Ad hoc training for visitors, focusing on listening skills and the role and responsibilities of the visitor, has been a feature of national provision in BCA, *ia* and UA in recent years. In a move to raise quality further and to ensure standards, *ia* is completing preparation to offer accredited training to its existing and would-be visitors. The intention is to ensure that the visit is handled, as it were, professionally and that the valuable resource of experiential knowledge is used in a professional manner.

Despite the prominent part played in the formation of these groups by professionals, there is no guarantee today, especially at a local level, that the same spirit of cooperation will be found between the individual active in the ostomy group and the professional. The associations have to acknowledge, as Gidron and Hasenfeld (1994) and Simpson (1996) have noted, that power and control lie with the public service. Where professionals are not fully ready to accept that complementary services can be offered, the onus is on the voluntary organisations to demonstrate not only the benefits of this but also their ability to work effectively alongside such professionals.

CONCLUSION

The ostomy groups discussed in this chapter have demonstrated their value to the ostomist for a number of years. They are able to provide a potent form of direct support to individuals in a situation that can be difficult to cope with. Individuals have gained great strength from membership of these organisations, not to mention valuable and practical information. Additionally, the associations provide a voice on behalf of the ostomists when their interests need to be furthered or simply protected. The value of this work depends on the commitment, focus and skills of those ostomists active in their association. It also depends, crucially, on support from the professionals involved in stoma care and surgery. This area has been characterised by strong positive relationships but it is for both sides to be aware that what exists needs maintaining and that there are areas where improvements would be welcome. For effective cooperation, both voluntary groups and professionals need to have an awareness of each other's situation and also to recognise they have a goal in common – the wellbeing of the ostomist.

REFERENCES

Alexander, N. (1998) *ia Journal* 163. *ia*.

Borkman, T. (1997) A selective look at self-help groups in the United States. *Health and Social Care in the Community;* 5: 6, 357–364.

Bottomley, A. (1997) Cancer support groups – are they effective? *European Journal of Cancer Care;* 6, 11–17.

Gidron, B., Hasenfeld, Y. (1994) Human service organisations and self-help groups: can they collaborate? *Non-profit Management and Leadership;* 5 (Winter 1994), 159–172.

Hildingh, C., Fridlund, B., Segesten, K. (1995) Social support in self-help groups, as experienced by persons having coronary heart disease and their next of kin. *International Journal of Nursing Studies;* 32: 3, 224–232.

Rootes, L., Aanes, D. (1992) A conceptual framework for understanding self-help groups *Hospital and Community Psychiatry;* 43: 4, 379–381.

Simpson, R. (1996) Relationships between self-help health organisations and professional health care providers. *Health and Social Care in the Community;* 4: 6, 359–370.

The Rising of the Phoenix: The Origins of *ia* (1996) *ia Midlands News Bulletin.*

9 Cultural issues

Fran Pinches

'A physician is obligated to consider more than a diseased organ, more even than the whole man – he must view the man in his world.'

Harvey Cushing (1869–1939) US Surgeon

It is not intended to give an in-depth and expert dissertation of worldwide religions and cultures, but more an opportunity to consider our patients as individuals and perhaps ponder why reactions to stoma surgery can be so varied. Each one of us has our own way of viewing and handling a situation, personal codes of behaviour and life values; does the way that we live our life simply happen, or do we as individuals reflect our parents' standards or perhaps our educational experiences? There would seem to be no categorical answer to that question, nor should there be in a society that is democratic and also becoming progressively multicultural.

Nursing care plans, although essentially similar, when completed will always differ due to the individual needs of the patient. It may be due to the illness, treatment, race, age, sex or even religion of the person involved. Certainly, each factor will in some way affect or be affected by one or more of the others.

The need for stoma surgery can present at any age and for a myriad of reasons. The stoma may be permanent or temporary, a planned procedure or the result of an emergency situation. The initial reaction to the stoma will most likely be one of dislike and possibly revulsion, but with good pre- and postoperative counselling and support most patients will learn to cope and begin their return to health and to their society successfully. Smith (1992) states that the preoperative period is a time when the patient and family are seeking information, dealing with the fear and anxiety of the unknown, and activating coping strategies.

In the western world stoma surgery has become accepted as the best surgical option for many conditions; bowel cancer and inflammatory bowel disease being amongst the most common. Although cancer is a worldwide problem inflammatory bowel disease is extremely uncommon in eastern and third world countries (Nicholls, 1998) but is becoming more prevalent in second and third generations of western ethnic communities. Being born and often educated in their adopted country the younger ethnic population, particularly Asian, is becoming more westernised in dress and lifestyle but their cultural upbringing is still often strictly adhered to. Religious education is given after school and practised in a traditional manner, often necessitating prayer several times during the day.

In the completion of care plans it is both lamentable and frustrating to often find in the 'Religion' section only one word noted. It seems that along with sexuality, religion is a subject not to be explored but one to be glossed over, perhaps to avoid embarrassment. Alternatively if the nurse concerned is of a different religion or is not fluent in the patient's language a difficulty in seeking further facts may be experienced. Assistance from relatives can be one solution, for example establishing any dietary restrictions – once considered the only special need for those of eastern faiths; how ignorant the British were 30 or 40 years ago!

Table 9.1 Possible difficulties

Language difficulty
Embarrassment
Belief in reincarnation

Obtaining basic information may be sufficient for those patients undergoing minor surgery but when altered body image will result counselling with relatives as interpreters is unsatisfactory. Discussion will, or should, include intimate details of the patient's feelings and fears and many people find difficulty in expressing themselves freely in the presence of close family. Most communities are able to provide help with translators and when there is limited written material available in the particular language or dialect such a service is vital in order to gain informed consent to treatment. Obtaining consent for surgery may need a family discussion, particularly concerning the female Asian patient (Sampson, 1982).

Agreement by the male elder of the family is still respected in the traditional family group and time should be allowed for this to avoid misunderstanding and delay in treatment.

THE MULTIRACIAL SOCIETY

Travel around the world is now commonplace giving rise to a multiracial society with a profusion of cultural and religious beliefs. Large towns and cities often boast Chinese, Vietnamese, Thai, Afro-Caribbean, Indian, Italian, Greek, and Jewish communities – so many immigrant groups are now well integrated into our communities. It is inevitable that at some time individuals from one or all of these communities will be treated by healthcare staff, and that for one reason or another an aspect of their culture will be of consequence.

Each religion has its own written scripture or text and the depth of conformity will vary from person to person. For example, several faiths state an expectation of 'perfection in the sight of God' which people have frequently interpreted as bodily perfection, causing great distress when a permanent stoma was decreed necessary. Discussing the term 'perfection' in reference to the way the patient lives their life rather than their physical appearance will often give reassurance and talking to their priest, minister, rabbi, imam or church elder may be helpful.

The subject of reincarnation can be looked at in a similar way. Belief that the body is only lent for the time spent on earth can be troublesome when facing what is, after all, mutilating surgery. Reincarnation is the belief of the Hindu, Sikh and Buddhist faiths; the cycle of birth and rebirth. Henley and Clayton (1982) note that the form in which you are reborn depends on your thoughts and actions in your previous life. The belief in karma – that ill fortune in the present life is due to a sinful previous existence – may have a profound psychological effect on the patient. An expected rejection by the family and community may result in depression and despondency with inevitable poor motivation to rehabilitate. Being able to include an understanding of possible concerns in preoperative counselling, however small, will possibly ease fears and initiate a better understanding between the nurse and the patient. It will most certainly demonstrate a caring philosophy within the department and a degree of empathy in unfamiliar surroundings.

PRACTICAL MANAGEMENT

Learning to care for a stoma is never easy either practically or psychologically and requires encouragement at every step. On seeing the stoma for the first time a person of any faith or even an agnostic will ask, 'Why me? What have I done to deserve this?' A sense of unfairness is common when faced with an unpleasant situation and must be handled with a positive sensitivity particularly when a belief in 'karma' is an inherent part of the patient's life. Aesthetically a stoma is at first unpleasant for the patient to observe and care for. It is much more difficult when a person's religion seems to obstruct the achievement of self-care and acceptance by their social group. The custom among many Muslims that the right hand is used only for eating and greeting (Sampson, 1982) and the left for cleansing (clean hand and dirty hand) is fairly well understood by many healthcare staff but needs special consideration when teaching stoma care. An appliance should be chosen that can be managed easily and competently with one hand while also being suitable for the type of output produced. There is no hard and fast rule but a choice should be offered between a one-piece and two-piece appliance.

Table 9.2 Preoperative considerations

Allow for family involvement
Possible need for consent by male family member
Advice from religious leader

CHOICE OF APPLIANCE

Choosing an appliance is a very personal matter and because it is to lie next to the skin can be likened to choosing one's underwear. All patients will need to feel comfortable with a pouch or bag that is as discreet as possible. Often this will be a modern one-piece appliance that is lightweight, flexible, invisible beneath clothing and that will need changing twice daily at most. For the patient practising a religion that demands prayer frequently each and every day further thought is essential. The devout Muslim will follow the laws of his faith to the letter, meaning that he will need to pray five times each day and perform ablutions prior to prayer. This may require removal of the stoma bag to be replaced with a clean one on each occasion. If a one-piece bag is used the peristomal skin would be at risk of excoriation and could be rather a trial for the person concerned. The number of bags used each month would also be prohibitive. A far better choice would be a two piece appliance with obvious benefits both to the patient and the NHS! Whitehead (1982) notes that the ensuing skin problems can be minimised by using a two–piece bag. This must be a secure appliance, particularly if prostration is required during prayer. For the patient with a permanent sigmoid colostomy the use of the colostomy plug or management by colostomy irrigation could also be a solution to the problem. Consent from the surgeon must be obtained for this style of management and both methods taught by a qualified stoma care nurse. Not all patients will follow their religious teachings so fastidiously and may be willing to accept exemption, which may be given in cases of illness or incapacity.

As in the West traditions can change but it is interesting to read in an article on stoma care in Malaya that having a stoma caused much soul searching for the mainly Islamic population. Tan Tang Peng (1996), a Malaysian stoma care nurse, was repeatedly asked during the 1980s how a person was to pray with an uncontrollable ostomy. 'The matter was discussed by the country's religious panel. A year later, a 'fatwa' (ruling) was issued: the ostomate may perform his religious duties after he has cleaned his bag. Any passage of flatus or faeces into the bag during prayer is considered religiously excused, as long as nothing leaks outside the bag.'

SITING THE STOMA

Most surgeons considered it the responsibility of the stoma care nurse to decide on a suitable site for the stoma. Stoma site selection must be a priority for the healthcare team (Smith, 1992). An improperly placed stoma complicates the patient's self-care and may have a negative effect on adaptation. Although there are guidelines to be followed, each patient's abdomen will present its own problem and detailed discussion is often required before a suitable site is agreed with the patient. It is generally accepted in western society that the stoma will be less obtrusive and troublesome at a site below the waistline thus avoiding waist and belt lines, which may cause leakage and possible trauma to the stoma. However, when the belief is such that food passing through the digestive tract is regarded as clean while it remains above the umbilicus but becomes waste material, and therefore dirty, below that point the rules must be allowed to bend.

When siting any stoma in a case of planned surgery the nurse must ensure that the patient is comfortable with the siting. Much will depend on the type of clothing worn: if western dress is worn then the patient may well prefer a lower siting and be willing to compromise. Discussion during preoperative counselling will enable the patient to consider this point and perhaps talk with family elders or religious leaders. Other than the initial acceptance of stoma surgery, siting is considered one of the vitally important areas of preoperative preparation, as poor siting can result in management problems along with psychological trauma.

INFORMED CONSENT

The signing of a consent form has been a thorn in the flesh over the past few years, seen by many patients simply as a document to be signed for receiving a general anaesthetic or giving the surgeon permission to carry out the planned procedure and anything else that he may need to do. Levels of comprehension will vary and it is vital that the patient's understanding is as full as possible. Allen (1998) states it is important that the nurse checks their understanding at each stage. In Britain a married couple will have no great difficulty in agreeing together that the surgery is acceptable, but in many ethnic groups a need to discuss the details with the family will be expressed. Often the male elder of the family will be consulted and his permission obtained, demonstrating the respect that the extended family has for its senior members. Indeed other family members find it quite difficult if it is the respected family elder who is the patient and is unable to give consent for himself, particularly when emergency stoma surgery may be in question. In this respect, of course, the Asian family is no different to any other but their tradition highlights the responsibility.

DIET AND NUTRITION

Correct nutrition is vital to recovery after any illness and is particularly important following intestinal surgery. Preoperative bowel preparation followed by intravenous infusion until the gut resumes its normal function frequently results in a patient with poor appetite and a fairly slow return to a normal eating pattern. For the patient with a newly formed stoma, beginning to eat solid food can be an anxious time. Although patients are advised to aim towards as normal a diet as possible they will have been advised that a high fibre diet may result in over production of flatus or loose stool. If the patient is not on a restricted diet for any other medical reasons a slight dietary adaptation should be no problem. Consider then the vegetarian of whom there are an increasing number, be it for religious or moral reasons. Some years ago being a vegetarian was considered by many to be slightly 'weird' or 'cranky' but gradually the right to avoid eating meat has become accepted. Whatever the reason for following a vegetarian diet, correct and timely advice is essential for both return to health and a good quality lifestyle.

Several of the eastern faiths require observance of dietary restriction but vary in stringency. The Hindu faith teaches that all living things are sacred and therefore Hindus have a strict vegetarian code, not eating meat, fish or even eggs. Sikhism being an offshoot of the Hindu faith bans beef and pork but allows some fish, chicken and eggs, although many choose to keep to a vegetarian diet. Followers of Islam are not allowed pork and any other meat must be killed by the Halal method. Fish is allowed but has to have fins, although seafood, such as lobster or crab, is not eaten. Orthodox Jews also will not eat fish without fins, pork or its products and will not have meat and milk products at the same meal. Many Orthodox Jews will require a vegetarian diet unless the meat (not pork) is 'Kosher', killed by a specially trained butcher. Rastafarians may also follow a vegetarian diet of varying strictness. Exceptionally strict Rastafarians will only eat food cooked in vegetable oil and some may not wish to eat in public.

Table 9.3 Practical aspects

Stoma siting
Use of one hand – clean hand/dirty hand
Dietary restrictions
Frequency of prayer – religious festivals

For the patient who is obviously malnourished an early referral to the dietician or specialist nutrition nurse should be routine and regular weight checks made. The patient with an ileostomy may become dehydrated if the output is very liquid and as well as dietary advice may need antidiarrhoea medication and careful follow-up. It is important that the patient should not feel that their diet is a problem to nursing staff, instead they should be encouraged and supported during a difficult period.

RELIGIOUS FESTIVALS

To discuss the multitude of religious festivals celebrated throughout the world would be quite impossible within this text and mostly irrelevant to the patient with a stoma, but those with implications for dietary restriction can present some difficulty for those patients. Festivals such as Ramadan and Yom Kippur, both of which involve fasting, are very special and although dispensation for the sick person may be given many will wish to observe the ritual unless their condition is poor. Christian festivals are not associated with fasting other than possibly during Lent, but the rich, high fibre foods eaten at Christmas may have disastrous consequences if a large amount is devoured over a short period. The old maxim of 'everything in moderation' is good advice with regard to celebration or devotion in any cultural observance.

CONCLUSION

The indigenous population of any country has its own culture and standards that are essential to the stability of its community. In the modern world almost every country sees a variety of peoples be it those on business, on holiday or living permanently in a country of their choice and for whatever reason. The old adage of 'when in Rome' can no longer be used as an excuse for ignoring the needs of those of other races or creeds. By the very nature of her role, the nurse in the community enjoys the very privileged status of being invited into patients' homes and seeing the patient as a family member rather than a sick individual during a stay in the rather alien environment of a hospital ward. The stoma care nurse is perhaps even more privileged as most are able to see the patient both in the hospital and the community. Patient confidentiality is an accepted part of professional nurse conduct but for the patient trust grows gradually out of respect for the nurse. The professional can generate a degree of empathy by actively demonstrating an understanding or a willingness to learn some of the customs and concerns of our ethnic population, thus helping the patient with an altered body image to accept their changed appearance and the early difficulties which no doubt will occur. It may be that the patient who is linked to a particular spiritual belief will not wish to receive any special consideration but it is important to demonstrate an understanding of individual differences. On reflection it may be that in living life within the law and respecting our own particular customs perhaps it is the similarities that outweigh the differences when considering cultural aspects surrounding stoma care. Nurses clearly need to be open-minded in their approach to this vital aspect of nursing care (Burnard and Chapman, 1998).

REFERENCES

Allen, S. (1998) Update. *Professional Nurse;* 14: 2.

Burnard, P, Chapman, C. (1988) *Professional and Ethical Issues in Nursing: The Code of Professional Conduct.* Chichester: John Wiley and Sons.

Henley, A., Clayton, J. (1982) Illness and the life cycle: Asians in hospital. *Health and Social Service Journal;* August, 972–973.

Nicholls, R.J. (1998) Ulcerative colitis in colorectal surgery. In: Phillips, R.K.S. (ed.) *Colorectal Surgery.* London: W.B. Saunders Co Ltd.

Peng, Tan Tang (1996) Ostomy care in Malaysia – A cultural view. *World Council of Enterostomal Therapists Journal;* 16: 1, 30–31.

Sampson, C. (1982) *The Neglected Ethic: Religious and Cultural Factors in the Care of Patients.* Maidenhead: McGraw-Hill Book Company (UK) Ltd.

Smith, D.B. (1992) Psychosocial adaptation. In: Hampton, B.J., Bryant, R.A. (eds.) *Ostomies and Continent Diversions: Nursing Management.* St. Louis, Missouri: Mosby.

Whitehead, M. (1981) Ostomists: A world of difference. *Journal of Community Nursing;* 4:10.

FURTHER READING

Sampson, C. (1982) *The Neglected Ethic: Religious and Cultural Factors in the Care of Patients.* Maidenhead: McGraw-Hill Book Company (UK) Ltd.

An easy-to-read book designed to encourage awareness of patients' backgrounds. An overall view of various worldwide religions and the cultural factors arising from them. Religions listed alphabetically for plucking out relevant facts quickly.

Burnard, P, Chapman, C. (1988) *Professional and Ethical Issues in Nursing: The Code of Professional Conduct.* Chichester: John Wiley and Sons.

Chapter 6 is devoted to customs, values and spiritual beliefs of patients/clients. It assists in reflection and encourages an open-minded approach to those with or without religious beliefs.

Fisher, M.P. (1997) *Living Religions: An Encyclopaedia of the World's Faiths.* London: I.B. Taurie Ltd.

A highly readable and stimulating survey of the modern religious world encompassing traditional faiths, indigenous religions and new religious movements. It focuses on the historical development and teachings of each religion and explores how these traditions have evolved into contemporary beliefs and practices.

The Hutchinson Encyclopaedia of Living Faiths. (1988) Zaehner, R.C. (ed.) 4th Edition. First published by Hutchinson Ltd 1959. Reprinted by Helicon Publishing Ltd 1993.

Designed as a reference for world religions, discussing religions and beliefs as well as major writings of each faith.

10 Stomal complications

Penny Taylor

> 'Volumes are now written and spoken upon the effect of the mind on the body – much of it true. But I wish a little more was thought of the effect of the body on the mind.'
>
> (Florence Nightingale, 1859)

From time to time problems directly related to the care of the stoma may occur. The following two chapters will cover some of the more common problems: the first looks at the problems in the stoma management and the second will look more in depth at the skin conditions that may arise due to the stoma and the wearing of a pouch.

A skin problem can occur at any time following stoma surgery and for a variety of reasons. When there is a skin problem it can be a very difficult time for the patient, and very trying and time-consuming for the multidisciplinary caring team. It is for this reason that an entire chapter of this book has been devoted to skin function and disorders.

As has been noted throughout this book, assessment is the key to the best plans and the optimum care should a problem arise. The stoma and the parastomal area need to be assessed but must be part of the greater sphere of holistic assessment and care.

There are several stomal problems to consider and they are described here.

POORLY SITED STOMA

A well sited stoma will give quality of life to the person with a stoma. A stoma should be positioned where the patient can see it. It could be said that if the person cannot see it they cannot be expected to correctly place a pouch over it for efficient collection of effluent. The stoma needs to be away from skin creases, bony prominences and scars; the waistline also needs to be avoided. It is usual to site the stoma within the rectus abdominus to reduce the incidence of herniation (Black, 1989; Kelly, 1995).

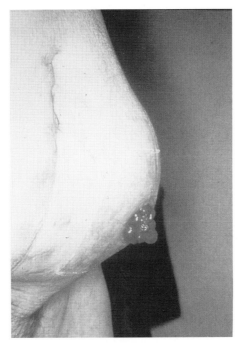

Fig 10.1 Patient unable to see the stoma.

Preoperative siting of a stoma is the most important physical care the stoma care nurse specialist can do for the patient. A well placed stoma is essential for quality of life; a poorly sited stoma can lead to many postoperative problems. These may include leakage and sore parastomal skin, which in turn can lead to social isolation and psychological problems for the patient.

NECROSIS

Necrosis can happen to a stoma in the early postoperative days. It will occur when there is a compromised blood supply to the bowel. The stoma may appear a dusky purple at first and then progress to black, a truly necrotic stoma.

The inadequate blood supply may be immediately postoperative due to difficulties during surgery, particularly if the patient has a large abdomen and mobilisation of the intestine perioperatively has been difficult. However, necrosis can occur later due to an ill fitting appliance.

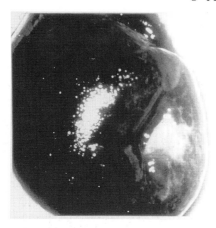

Fig 10.2

STENOSIS

Stenosis is the narrowing of the lumen or outlet of the stoma. Stenosis may be due to scar tissue, which can form around the stoma if separation of the mucocutaneous junction occurs during the immediate postoperative period, or if severe infection occurs. Scar tissue will be laid down if necrosis has been partial and sloughed away; healing then takes place. Scar tissue does not have the elasticity of normal tissue, so a stenosis occurs. These stomas will usually require surgical intervention.

RETRACTION

A retracted stoma usually means that it is no longer visible on the abdominal wall – it is sunken or it is in a dip. This may be due to poor healing at the mucocutaneous junction and the stoma slipping back. Later it may be due to weight gain. These stomas can be managed with an appropriate appliance and accessory products. Advice should be sought from the local specialist stoma care nurse.

PROLAPSE

A prolapsed stoma can be defined when a length of bowel prolapses out onto the exterior of the abdominal wall. This may be seen in any stoma but it is more common in transverse loop colostomies. Stoddart (1996) describes a 20% incidence of prolapsing transverse loop colostomy in her study.

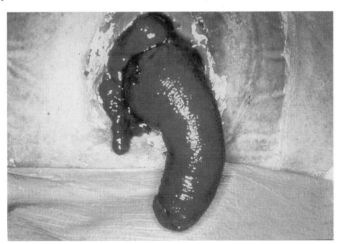

Fig 10.3

This condition can be very frightening for the patient who will need careful explanation of what is happening and a lot of reassurance. Stoma management can be difficult and the patient may need to be taught to reduce the prolapse in order to apply a pouch. However, it is not always possible to do this and the patient will need further advice on stoma management.

HERNIATION

A parastomal hernia is an abnormal amount of intestine in the subcutaneous or interstitial tissues and may occur with any stoma. The size and degree of herniation varies greatly from patient to patient. The hernia in an older person may be larger than in a younger person due to the loss of muscle tone in the older age group.

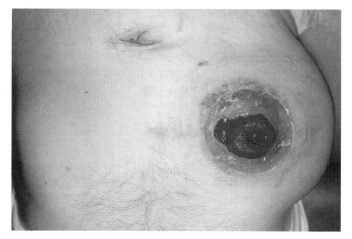

Fig 10.4 Herniation and sore skin due to an incorrect size of pouch

When a hernia occurs it is of concern to the patient. They not only feel they have to wear a pouch that may be seen (in their view) as a 'bulge' under clothing, but now they have a definite bulge that can be noticed under clothing. One option for management is to have further surgery to repair the hernia, but this carries no guarantee of success. A less invasive method of management is to wear an abdominal support garment. Everingham (1998) discusses the dilemma of parastomal hernia management in her paper and considers that more evidence-based nursing practice is needed in this area.

TRAUMA TO THE STOMA

Fortunately trauma to the stoma is not frequently seen, but does need to be considered along with the other stoma problems. Trauma may result from multiple injuries due to a road traffic accident or other major trauma incident.

More usually, injury or trauma to a stoma is caused by an ill-fitting pouch. The diameter of the aperture of the pouch is too small for the circumference of the stoma and in fitting the pouch the stoma is traumatised. This is usually in the form of a laceration.

The management of this condition is to fit a correctly sized pouch, along with patient education, so as to prevent this happening again. The lacerated area will heal quickly once the problem is removed.

During my career in stoma care nursing I have had one case of self-inflicted trauma to the stoma. This is not something that can be diagnosed lightly. It is something that becomes apparent only after recurrent visits and the use of the counselling skills of the multidisciplinary team. People who are self-harming need sensitive and expert help.

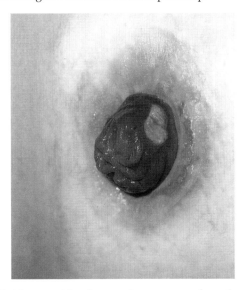

Fig 10.5 Ulcer on side of stoma due to trauma from the pouch

BLEEDING

The visual part of the stoma is the mucus membrane lining of either the small intestine or the colon. This tissue has a good natural blood supply. When cleansing the stoma some blood may appear on the cleansing tissue. This is normal and the patient needs to be made aware of this. However, the patient needs to also be aware that if bleeding occurs from the centre of the stoma it should be reported to their doctor in the same way as one would if bleeding occurs per rectum.

'PANCAKING'

This term is used to describe a situation when colostomy effluent does not fall to the bottom of the pouch but remains at the top and around the stoma. This can be uncomfortable for the patient and may also cause leakage between the pouch and the parastomal skin. The filter in the pouch can block and allow odour to leak from the pouch. If left unchecked the patient can become distressed due to the release of the odour and sore skin.

Pancaking occurs due to the pouch filter functioning normally and releasing all the air from the pouch, thus creating a vacuum inside. The pouch sides adhere to each other forming an obstruction to the flow of faeces.

The methods of management are:

▶ Use of pouch filter cover. This can be removed when the pouch begins to fill.

▶ A small tissue placed in the bottom of the pouch before application.

▶ Some Vaseline or similar product smeared inside the pouch before the application.

Alleviating the problem will prevent sore skin.

ODOUR

Odour and the fear of smelling are of paramount importance to the patient. When told they need to have a stoma formed one of the first questions they ask is, 'Will I smell?'.

If the patient complains of smelling or the family/carer smells a malodour this needs to be investigated. Points to consider are:

- Personal hygiene regarding pouch and stoma management. If a drainable pouch is used it may be that the patient is not cleaning the outlet well and the residual effluent is causing the odour.

- Pouch leakage.

- Leakage and/or blockage of the filter. Odour can also occur if the pouch is not put on correctly; there may be small creases in the adhesive part of the pouch.

- Dietary intake (see Chapter 12).

Having made the assessment, an action plan can be put into place to relieve the problem. The use of deodorant sprays may be helpful. There is a wide range available now either 'over the counter' or on prescription.

FISTULAE

Sometimes a fistula may form next to the stoma. This is usually in a patient with a diagnosis of Crohn's disease. This condition frequently requires surgical intervention.

ALTERATION IN BOWEL HABIT

For people with an ileostomy or colostomy a change in the normal output to their stoma may occur. This may be an increase or a decrease in output. If a patient complains of a change in habit this should be addressed and the following points considered:

- What is the usual bowel habit?

- What has it changed to?

▶ Has there been a change in any of the following?

- Diet
- Drugs
- Mobility
- Finances
- Mouth care
- Fluid intake
- Recurrent or new pathology

(Winney, 1998)

Only when an assessment has been made can a plan of care be made.

The use of enemas and suppositories has little effect in the management of constipation in a patient with a colostomy. A colostomy has no sphincters so they will be expelled immediately from the bowel.

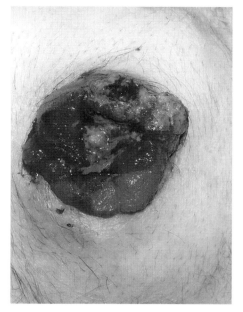

Fig 10.6 Recurrence of carcinoma on the stoma

URINARY TRACT INFECTION

Patients with an ileal conduit/urostomy have a shortened urinary tract system, and can be susceptible to recurrent urine infections. As part of the patient assessment a urine specimen may need to be taken for culture. This specimen should not be collected from the pouch. Guidelines for the collection of a urine specimen can be found in the Royal Marsden Hospital Manual of Clinical Nursing Procedures (1999).

Points to consider when giving advice would be:

▶ Patient's personal hygiene, stoma care management and management of the night drainage system.

▶ Fluid intake, with the introduction of cranberry juice. Cranberry juice used in a study by Rogers (1991) was shown to reduce the incidence of urinary tract infections in patients with indwelling catheters. This is also applicable to patients with a stoma.

CONCLUSION

As previously stated in this chapter, the key to problem solving is the assessment. If assessment takes place management systems can be put in place to resolve the patient's problem. The easier stoma management is for the patient the less potential there is of psychological morbidity and social isolation for this patient group.

REFERENCES

Black, P.K. (1989) Complications associated with a stoma. *Surgical Nurse;* 2: 6, Supplement I–v.

Everingham, L. (1998) The parastomal hernia dilemma. *World Council of Enterostomal Therapy Journal;* 18: 1, 32–34.

Kelly, L. (1995) Patients becoming people. *Journal of Community Nursing;* August 12–16.

Rogers, J. (1991) Pass the cranberry juice. *Nursing Times;* 87: 48.

Stoddart, M. (1996) Research into the incidence and management of prolapsed loop colostomy. *Proceedings of 11th Biennial Congress of the World Council of Enterostomal Therapists;* June 1996, 123–126.

Mallet, J., Bailey, C. (eds.) (1999) *The Royal Marsden NHS Trust Manual Of Clinical Nursing Procedures.* 4th Edition. Oxford: Blackwell Science.

Winney, J. (1998) Constipation. *Nursing Standard;* 13: 11, 49–56.

FURTHER READING

Elcoat, C. (1986) *Stoma Care Nursing.* London: Bailière Tindall.

Myers, C. (ed.) (1996) *Stoma Care Nursing: A Patient Centred Approach.* London: Arnold.

11 Skin disorders

Callum Lyon

As many as two-thirds of stoma patients experience a skin problem for which they consult their stoma nurse or general practitioner. This high prevalence of skin disease is to be expected given the abnormal stresses to which the skin is subjected under a stoma appliance. These stresses are occlusion, maceration, irritation and shearing forces for which the skin of the abdomen is not adapted. These factors will increase the likelihood of infection, allergy and irritant dermatitis. There are, in addition, several pre-existing skin disorders that appear at sites of skin damage and can cause problems around stomas, psoriasis being the most frequent.

In this chapter I will describe the structure of the skin, its response to trauma, irritants and allergens and discuss the variety of skin diseases seen in stoma patients.

ANATOMY AND PHYSIOLOGY OF THE SKIN

The skin is not merely a physical barrier between the individual and the external environment; it also serves metabolic, communication and homeostatic functions (Table 11.1). Knowledge of the skin's structure (Fig 11.1), repair mechanisms and protective responses is useful in understanding the disease processes seen around stomas.

Table 11.1 Functions of the skin

Function	Skin structure involved
Communication	
sensation	sensory nerves: pain, temperature, touch, vibration
flushing	blood vessels under nervous control
body odour	apocrine sweat glands in axillae, groins, nipples
Metabolism	
vitamin D synthesis	keratinocytes
energy storage	subcutaneous fat
Regulatory	
temperature	blood vessels under nervous control
	eccrine sweat glands
prevention of water, electrolyte and protein loss	horny layer
Protective	
physical	
chemical	horny layer and sebum secretion
trauma	horny layer
ultraviolet light	horny layer and melanocytes
immunological	langerhans cells

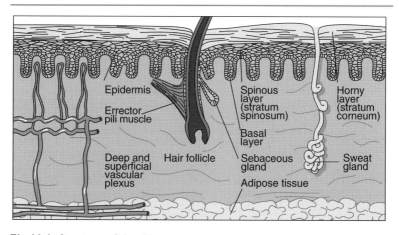

Fig 11.1 Structure of the skin

The skin consists of two layers: the epidermis and the underlying dermis. The epidermis is formed from many layers of cells called keratinocytes, which produce keratin proteins. It ranges in thickness from 0.1mm on eyelids to 1mm on palms and soles. The cells are continually produced by division of the cells in the basal layer. As the cells progress up to the surface they first form the spinous layer where cells are firmly held together by protein bonds. In the next layer, the granular layer, the cells have differentiated to become flatter and contain abundant keratin proteins. As the cells move on to the horny layer (stratum corneum) they lose their nuclei and essentially become a stack of flat, dead cells which acts as a protective, waterproof barrier layer. The time from basal layer to surface (approximately 60 days) and the thickness of the epidermis are tightly regulated by signalling proteins, including cytokines, and growth factors. These mechanisms respond to the environment so that the keratin layer may become thickened as a protective response to repeated pressure or rubbing, for example to form callosities.

In addition to keratinocytes the epidermis contains other important cells and structures. Melanocytes produce melanin pigments, which are injected in packets into neighbouring basal keratinocytes where they serve to protect the DNA in the nucleus from ultraviolet light damage. Langerhans cells are bone marrow derived cells, which play an important role in immunological surveillance and protection. They take up antigens (chemicals which stimulate an immunological response), either microbial proteins or other chemicals, process them and present them to T-lymphocytes. The latter will then orchestrate a protective, immunological response against microbial attack. Unfortunately the system occasionally generates a response to harmless antigens and results in allergic contact dermatitis. The commonest are nickel and fragrances, although several of the chemicals used in manufacturing appliances such as stoma pouches have also been reported to cause allergy by this mechanism.

The epidermis also contains the eccrine sweat glands that produce sweat under the control of autonomic nerves. Sweat contains ammonia and urea and is acidic (pH 4–6.8), so that as well as a temperature control function sweat may discourage the overgrowth of some pathogenic bacteria. The sebaceous glands produce greasy secretions that waterproof the skin and may also limit the proliferation of certain bacteria and fungi. These glands are usually associated with a hair follicle, but around the eyes, mouth, anus and genitalia they occur independently and may be abundant.

The dermis and epidermis are held firmly together by strong collagen protein fibres. Where the epidermis and dermis meet, interlocking projections from both surfaces serve to increase the surface area for adhesion. The principal cell of the dermis is the fibroblast, which produces the collagen, elastic fibres and ground substance that together make up the bulk of the dermis. The dermis contains the network of blood vessels, lymphatics and nerves.

Response of the skin to injury

When the skin is subjected to repeated mild trauma from rubbing, scraping, chemical irritation or strong sunlight there is a protective response to increase the thickness of the keratin layer. This produces calluses, commonly seen on the hands and feet. In itchy skin diseases where there is inflammation, such as eczema, repeated scratching or rubbing results in thickened leathery skin (lichenification). Such responses are achieved through the regulatory action of local growth factors and cytokines on keratinocyte proliferation.

Acute cutting, heat or chemical damage produces repair responses. If the damage is superficial, involving only the epidermis or upper dermis, the epidermis can regrow from the edges and from the epithelial lining of hair follicles to cover the defect without scar formation. Deeper wounds heal with scars. In larger wounds where there is loss of tissue, the resulting scar contracts to reduce the size of the defect (secondary intention wound). In surgical incisions the edges are held together with sutures and there is no contraction of the scar (primary intention wound). In all deeper skin wounds, where there is blood vessel damage and haemorrhage, haemostasis is achieved via the clotting protein cascades and the aggregation of platelets that plugs holes in the vessels. Signalling proteins including growth factors and chemo-attractants are released by platelets and damaged skin cells. Together with a local nerve reflex, these serve to increase blood flow to the injured areas and promote leakage of fluid. This causes the redness and swelling seen in acute inflammation. The chemo-attractant proteins cause an influx of white blood cells, initially neutrophils. These cells begin to clear the wound area by phagocytosis of bacteria and other foreign particles. The other white cells entering the injured area are monocytes, which are then activated to become macrophages. These cells also release growth factors that stimulate the formation of granulation tissue; so called because of the fine, granular appearance of newly formed capillary blood vessels seen in healing wounds. The new blood vessels proliferate allowing a route for nutrients and inflammatory cells into the healing tissue. Fibroblasts are active producing collagen and ground substance proteins, providing the framework for the healing scar tissue. As wound repair progresses new vessel formation ceases and the number of new vessels diminishes.

Wound healing processes occasionally go wrong and the two commonest aberrations are of particular interest to stoma care. First, granulation tissue may proliferate rather than regressing and so produces over-granulation, sometimes called 'proud-flesh'. These tender red plaques bleed very easily and are readily treated by cautery or excision. Second, scarring may become very prominent, producing an irregular skin surface. Where the scar, although prominent, is within the area of skin which was injured, it is called a hypertrophic scar. Sometimes scar tissue extends laterally beyond the wound edge and can do so progressively. This is termed a keloid scar and these occur more commonly in darker skinned races.

SKIN DISORDERS IN STOMA PATIENTS

In this section I will describe the common and important rarer skin diseases seen around stomas. The figures quoted refer to my experience of a large number of ostomates with skin problems, seen in a joint clinic with a stoma care department. The majority of skin diseases (dermatoses) seen in stoma patients fall into the following broad categories:

- irritant reactions;

- pre-existing dermatoses;

- infections;

- parastomal ulceration;

- allergy.

These will be discussed in turn. Malignancies, usually metastatic spread from bowel or urinary carcinoma, occur occasionally around stomas and will not be discussed.

Irritant reactions

Ileostomies and colostomies: faecal irritant dermatitis

Irritant dermatitis from persistent contact with faeces is common (20% of ostomates with skin problems). Gut enzymes, particularly proteases and amylase cause faecal irritant dermatitis. It has been shown that, even at the rectum of normal individuals, the level of these small bowel enzymes is sufficient to cause irritant reactions (Andersen et al, 1994). The digestive effect of the enzymes and the occlusion of the stoma appliance combine to damage the barrier function of the horny layer of the skin and promote an inflammatory reaction. The epidermis may respond by thickening to produce the clinical appearance of lichenification. Faecal irritant reactions are seen more frequently around ileostomies than colostomies because the faeces produced at an ileostomy are more fluid and contain higher concentrations of digestive enzymes.

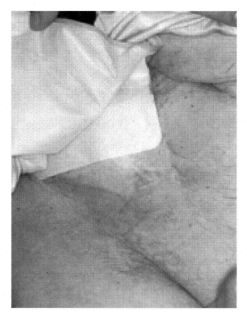

Fig 11.2 Leakage of faeces resulting from a colostomy sited in a scarred abdominal skin crease and leading to faecal irritant dermatitis extending from the stoma to the inguinal crease.

Leakage of faeces onto the skin is more likely with suboptimal stoma siting in an abdominal skin fold (Fig 11.2), or if the stoma is receding. In addition, the size of a stoma may change in the postoperative period so that the aperture in a stoma pouch barrier becomes too large allowing contact between skin and faeces. This results in a crescent shaped area of irritant dermatitis below the stoma. Occasionally patients may pick at their stoma pouch, by habit or because of a psychiatric disorder, and cause leakage resulting in dermatitis.

Urostomies

A poorly sited or receding stoma can also result in dermatitis from the effect on skin barrier function of prolonged contact with urine and the consequent maceration. A unique form of irritant reaction, termed chronic papillomatous dermatitis, may also be seen in urostomy patients, particularly those with receding stomas (Bergman et al, 1979). It presents as a crop of warty prominences around the stoma (Fig 11.3).

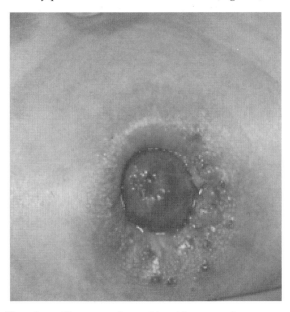

Fig 11.3 Chronic papillomatous dermatitis arising around a urostomy. The urostomy is recessed in abdominal fat resulting in leakage which causes this form of irritant dermatitis.

These may be itchy and occasionally painful. The warty areas result from local thickening of the epidermis and increased keratin production as a protective response to irritation. Stoma pouch adhesion can be impaired because of the irregular skin surface and this leads to further urine leakage and the potential for more lesions. It is important to distinguish this condition from simple viral warts and skin carcinoma in order to avoid inappropriate treatment and patient anxiety. In mild cases a convex backed bag prevents further leakage and the lesions resolve over a few weeks with no other treatment. In more extensive cases other measures, such as temporary catheterisation of the ileal conduit, may be necessary to rest the skin and allow recovery.

Over-granulation

As described above, this can occur in any healing wound. However, it can appear suddenly, many years after surgery, probably as a reaction to irritation. Around the stoma it is more commonly seen at the junction between skin and bowel but may occur in normal skin away from the stoma (Fig 11.4). Work with a small group of patients indicates that light freezing with liquid nitrogen spray is a more effective treatment than silver nitrate cautery and reduces the likelihood of recurrence.

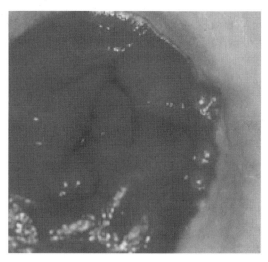

Fig 11.4 Papules of over-granulation at the junction between stoma and skin. These papules may be tender and bleed easily resulting in leaks.

Irritation from stoma materials

Chemical irritant dermatitis might occur to several of the constituents of stoma equipment. These include alcohol in wipes and pastes, karaya in pastes or barriers and the constituents of some adhesives. However, apart from two studies looking at adhesives and barriers (Marks et al, 1978; Burt-McAliley et al, 1994) little has been published on irritant dermatitis in stoma patients. Consequently the true incidence and individual causes are not yet known.

Pre-existing skin disease

Over 2,000 skin diseases are described in textbooks of dermatology most of which are very rare or uncommon. In theory most could occur around stomas and there are several individual case reports of uncommon diseases at this site (Vande Maele and Reilly, 1997; Rodriguez, 1981). The features of the more common skin disorders that occur around stomas will be discussed here.

Many dermatoses are generalised with features at several skin sites. It is therefore important to ask and to examine for skin disease elsewhere when assessing a patient with a parastomal rash as this may provide useful clues to the diagnosis. Patients presenting with these generalised conditions warrant referral to a dermatologist, as do any patients with unexplained or persistent skin disorders restricted to parastomal skin.

Psoriasis

Some dermatoses are more likely to be seen at sites of skin trauma (Koebner phenomenon). This is particularly true of psoriasis, one of the more common skin diseases with a prevalence in the general population of 1–3%. As a result one might expect to see it more frequently on the skin around stomas, and psoriasis has emerged as a particular problem, occurring around the stoma in 11% of patients who report a skin problem. There is a well recognised association between psoriasis and inflammatory bowel disease (Yates et al, 1982) and it appears that psoriasis is more common in patients with severe bowel disease that necessitates bowel surgery. Psoriasis is characterised by well demarcated, scaly red plaques, particularly on the elbows, knees, scalp and sacrum (Fig 11.5). It may also cause pitting or lifting of the nails and is occasionally associated with a generalised arthritis. In flexures such as the axilla and around stomas the plaques have a uniform, glazed red appearance (Fig 11.6).

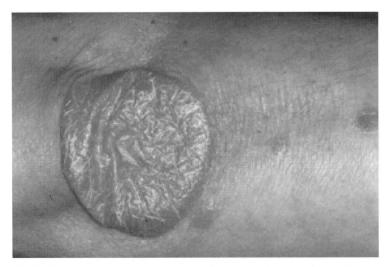

Fig 11.5 A typical plaque of psoriasis affecting the elbow. Note the discrete edge and silvery scale.

These may be itchy or sore and in parastomal lesions exudate can impair bag adhesion. Most cases of parastomal psoriasis respond rapidly to topical steroid in an alcohol-based lotion that does not interfere with bag adhesion. The occasional patient has severe parastomal or generalised psoriasis which warrants systemic or inpatient treatment.

Seborrhoeic dermatitis

This common skin disease may present around the stoma with a rash very similar to psoriasis. Like psoriasis it may also cause scaling and redness of the scalp but the other manifestations are distinct. These include fine, scaling erythema on the forehead, eyebrows, sides of the nose, chin and sometimes central chest. Whilst the cause of this condition is controversial it probably involves an inflammatory reaction to human commensal yeasts. Although it does respond to topical corticosteroid lotions it is perhaps better treated with an antifungal cream (imidazole) if the patient is able to wear a non-adhesive pouch.

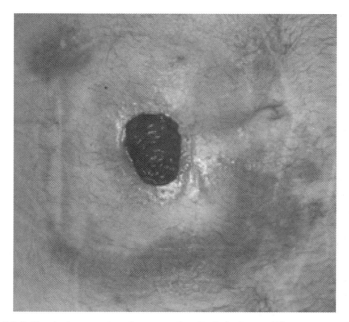

Fig 11.6 Psoriasis around an ileostomy for Crohn's disease. The upper patch is scaly whilst those under the stoma bag adhesive are glazed red in appearance.

Eczemas

The term eczema is derived from the Greek word for boiling and it refers to a florid red, exudative rash, often associated with tiny vesicles that give a bubbling appearance to the skin. Eczema is extremely common, accounting for around 5% of all general practice consultations. The vast majority of dermatologists use the terms 'dermatitis' and 'eczema' synonymously although dermatitis is perhaps used more frequently to describe allergic rashes, as in the term 'allergic contact dermatitis' which will be discussed later.

Atopic eczema usually presents before one year of age with weeping, red areas of skin in the elbow and knee flexures, hands, feet and face. It may become generalised and is typically associated with asthma or hayfever. Discoid eczema presents with itchy, round, weeping areas usually on the legs of older men. These two types of eczema together account for only around 3% of parastomal skin problems. They both respond very well to topical steroid lotions. However, in resistant cases there may be secondary infection driving the inflammation, particularly with *Staphylococcus aureus*. For this reason it is important to swab inflamed eczematous rashes around stomas for microbiological examination. If infection is strongly suspected treatment with an oral antibiotic, such as flucloxacillin, is recommended before infection is confirmed.

Rare skin diseases

There are several uncommon, hereditary and acquired skin disorders which might cause parastomal skin problems.

The ichthyoses are scaling skin diseases that result from genetically abnormal keratins or failure of separation of cells in the horny layer. They produce dry, scaly skin that might interfere with bag adhesion.

Blistering skin diseases may result from genetically abnormal cell adhesion between keratinocytes or between the dermis and epidermis (epidermolysis bullosa). They may also be caused by autoimmune mechanisms where antibodies are directed against cell adhesion molecules. In each case the skin is likely to develop blisters at sites of trauma and problems have been described in stoma patients (Vande Maele and Reilly, 1997; Readding, 1998; Nemoto, 1998).

Infections

The warm, humid conditions under a stoma pouch are ideal for the growth of potentially pathogenic micro-organisms. Viral, bacterial and fungal infections account for 10% of skin problems in stoma patients.

Primary skin infections

These include the more common viral, bacterial and fungal infections (see Table 11.2).

Table 11.2 Common skin infections

Function	Skin manifestation
Viral	
Papilloma virus	Viral warts which may be confused with chronic papillomatous dermatitis.
Pox virus	Molluscum contagiosum – small pearly papules with a central depression. Usually affects children.
Herpes viruses	Cold sores – clusters of small blisters that recur at the same site.
Fungal	
Dermatophytes (ringworm)	Scaly, moist red rash with a distinct edge (Fig 11.7) and characteristic sour odour.
Candida	Itchy, confluent, red rash with surrounding smaller spots (satellites).
Pityrosporun	Blotchy, orange-pink rash or folliculitis.
Bacterial	
Staphylococcus	Impetigo – areas of superficial erosion with honey-coloured exudate and crust. Streptococci may also be involved.
	Folliculitis.
	Ecthyma – crusted ulceration that heals with scarring.
Streptococcus	Cellulitis – spreading infection in the deeper skin and subcutaneous tissues, producing a painful, red, oedematous area.
Diphtheroids (overgrowth of skin commensals)	Erythrasma – scaly, pink-orange patches in flexures.

Opportunistic infections

Because of the favourable environment under a stoma appliance, normally harmless commensal organisms may proliferate. These include Candida and Pityrosporun yeasts or diphtheroid bacteria discussed in Table 11.2. If the skin is broken, for example surgically or traumatically, the wound may become secondarily infected with skin pathogens, such as Streptococci or bowel pathogens such as Pseudomonas. This may produce purulent ulceration or spreading cellulitis, which requires specific, systemic antimicrobial therapy.

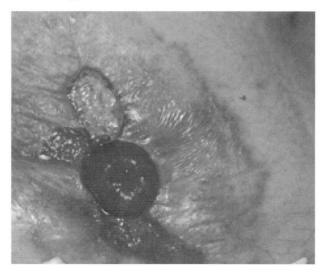

Fig 11.7 Tinea infection around a stoma. Note the faint red rash with a clearly-defined raised red border. The three areas of sloughing ulceration around the ileostomy in this patient with Crohn's disease are coincidental pyoderma gangrenosum.

Patients receiving chemotherapy or radiotherapy for malignancy or immunosuppressive therapy for inflammatory bowel disease are more susceptible to infection including skin infections. If a patient receiving one of these treatments presents with a new parastomal rash, they should be rapidly and carefully screened for infection.

Eczematous rashes and infection

It is now well recognised that staphylococcal skin infection can exacerbate eczema causing localised plaques to become generalised. This is because certain bacterial proteins termed superantigens may directly trigger a florid inflammatory response by binding to a receptor on white blood cells. For this reason most eczematous rashes should be swabbed for microbiological examination.

It has been suggested that some eczematous rashes around stomas are the result of allergy to one of several bacteria that may colonise parastomal skin (Anawaza, 1994). The evidence for this is very poorly described. However, the observation in small numbers of patients that some of these rashes will resolve with short courses of specific antibiotics warrants further investigation.

Parastomal ulceration

Ulceration around the stoma can severely affect a patient's lifestyle as a result of the pain and poor bag adhesion. The potential causes of persisting ulceration are listed in Table 11.3.

Table 11.3 Causes of persistent parastomal ulceration

Infection
> Synergistic gangrene
> Ecthyma (see Table 11.2)
> Syphilis
> Mycobacterial
> Fungal

Malignancy
> Secondary spread from colonic or urinary tract carcinoma
> Primary squamous carcinoma of the skin

Autoimmune
> Vasculitis
> Antiphospholipid antibody syndrome

Iatrogenic
> Radiotherapy related skin damage

Pyoderma gangrenosum

Associated diseases include:
> Inflammatory bowel disease
> Leukaemia, lymphoma and myeloma
> Wegener's granulomatosis

Pyoderma gangrenosum

Pyoderma gangrenosum (PG) is a rare, ulcerative skin condition of unknown cause that may be associated with systemic disease in up to 50% of cases (see Table 11.3). It is characterised by a painful ulcer with an undermined, purplish edge and purulent base (Fig 11.8). The diagnosis is a clinical one and is made when the other potential causes have been excluded. Although rare in general dermatology, PG appears to be the most common cause of persisting parastomal ulceration, perhaps because of the association with inflammatory bowel disease. Therapy relies on non-specific immunomodulatory drugs, such as corticosteroids, dapsone and cyclosporin. PG may resolve with topical corticosteroids. Ointments and creams are impractical for parastomal PG because of bag adhesion. Alcohol-based preparations are painful to apply but can be put on the pouch barrier and the alcohol allowed to evaporate before applying. This approach is particularly successful for shallower ulcers. Deeper ulcers often require systemic therapies under the supervision of a dermatologist. Intralesional injection of steroid has been reported to be effective in the treatment of PG. However, PG ulcers may respond to the trauma of injection by rapidly enlarging (pathergy phenomenon). In my experience this has occurred in three out of six patients injected, so intralesional injections are probably contraindicated.

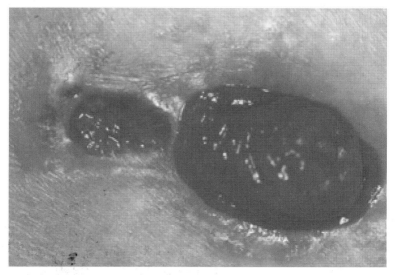

Fig 11.8 Pyoderma gangrenosum. The raised violaceous edge of this painful ulcer is typical. The patient has Crohn's disease.

Allergy

Despite the many potential causes of parastomal rashes described above, allergy is the one most patients and many health professionals first suspect. As a result patients have often tried a large variety of different stoma appliances by the time they present to a dermatologist. It is therefore surprising that apart from a few case reports describing allergy to substances in stoma equipment (Beck et al, 1985; O'Brien, 1986; van Hecke and Vossaert, 1988) there is little published on the subject.

The allergic response to antigens penetrating the skin involves the mechanisms described previously (langerhans cell and T-lymphocytes) and is called 'delayed type' because signs appear 48–72 hours after contact with the allergens. This type of allergy causes an eczematous rash usually called 'allergic contact dermatitis'. When the diagnosis is suspected it is investigated by patch testing, which involves the application of controlled concentrations of different chemicals to the patient's back under small adhesive dressings. These are removed two days later and any reactions are recorded. In stoma patients it is more likely that allergic contact dermatitis, when it does occur, is due to fragrances or preservatives in topical preparations rather than to the constituents of stoma pouches themselves. However, until a large patch testing study of all stoma patients with a rash is completed the true incidence of contact allergy and the allergens involved will remain unknown.

REFERENCES

Anawaza, S. (1994) Acute peristomal dermatitis caused by skin barrier: a form of bacterial allergy? Proceedings of the 10th Biennial Congress of the World Council of Enterostomal Therapists. *WCET*; 142–143.

Andersen, P.H., Bucher, A.P., Saeed, I. et al (1994) Faecal enzymes: in vivo human skin irritation. *Contact Dermatitis*; 30: 3, 152–158.

Beck, M.H., Burrows, D., Fregert, S. et al (1985) Allergic contact dermatitis to epoxy resin in ostomy bags. *British Journal of Surgery*; 72: 3, 202–203.

Bergman, B., Knutson, F., Lincoln, K. et al (1979) Chronic papillomatous dermatitis as a peristomal complication in conduit urinary diversion. *Scandinavian Journal of Urology and Nephrology*; 13: 2, 201–204.

Burt–McAliley, D., Eberhardt, D., van Rijswijk, L. (1994) Clinical study: peristomal skin irritation in colostomy patients. *Ostomy Wound Management;* 40: 6, 28–30, 32–34, 36–37.

Marks, R., Evans, E., Clarke, T.K. (1978) The effects on normal skin of adhesives from stoma appliances. *Current Medical Research and Opinion;* 5: 9, 720–725.

Nemoto, H. (1998) Management of pemphigoid at colostomy. Proceedings of the 12th Biennial Congress of the World Council of Enterostomal Therapists. *WCET;* 243–245.

O' Brien, T.J. (1986) Contact dermatitis to epoxy resin in ileostomy bag. *Australasian Journal of Dermatology;* 27: 2, 94–95.

Readding, L.A. (1998) Pemphigus: an experience. Proceedings of the 12th Biennial Congress of the World Council of Enterostomal Therapists. *WCET;* 187–189.

Rodriguez, D.B. (1981) Treatment for three ostomy patients with systemic skin disorders: psoriasis, pemphigus and dermatomyositis. *Journal of Enterostomal Therapy;* 8: 5, 31–32.

Vande Maele, D.M., Reilly, J.C. (1997) Bullous pemphigoid at colostomy site: report of a case. *Diseases of the Colon and Rectum;* 40: 3, 370–371.

van Hecke, E., Vossaert, K. (1988) Allergic contact dermatitis from an ostomy bag. *Contact Dermatitis;* 18: 2, 121–122.

Yates, V.M., Watkinson, G., Kelman, A. (1982) Further evidence for an association between psoriasis, Crohn's disease and ulcerative colitis. *British Journal of Dermatology;* 106: 3, 323–330.

FURTHER READING

General dermatology

Hunter, J.A.A., Savin, J.A., Dahl, M.V. (1995) *Clinical Dermatology.* Oxford: Blackwell Science.

Detailed text on dermatology and skin physiology

Fitzpatrick, T.B., Eisen, A.Z., Wolff, K. et al (1993) *Dermatology in General Medicine* (4th edition). New York: McGraw-Hill Inc.

12 Dietary considerations

Susan E. Bridgwater

Many people change their diet after having a stoma. The foods most often excluded are fruit and vegetables that are believed to cause embarrassing social problems, such as rapid filling of the bag, abdominal discomfort, wind or odour. So is it possible for ostomates to have a healthy, balanced diet?

DIGESTION AND ABSORPTION

The average time taken for food to pass along the gastrointestinal tract is one to three days. Digestion begins in the mouth as food is chewed and mixed with saliva. Food is then swallowed and passed down the oesophagus into the stomach. Here, food is mixed with hydrochloric acid, other gastric juices and intrinsic factor (necessary for vitamin B12 absorption).

A few substances are absorbed directly from the stomach including alcohol, water, glucose and certain minerals. Food is churned to a liquid in the stomach and remains there for around one to three hours. A low fibre carbohydrate meal would leave the stomach more quickly than a meal high in fibre, fat or protein and stomach clearing is more rapid when an individual is under emotional stress.

Liquidised food or chyme is then squirted intermittently into the small intestine. The small intestine is approximately three metres long and two to four centimetres in diameter (MAFF, 1995). Bile fluid and pancreatic juices are secreted to emulsify fat, neutralise the acid chyme from the stomach and digest fat, protein and carbohydrate. Absorption takes place along the whole of the small intestine. Vitamin B12, bound to intrinsic factor has special absorption sites only at the terminal ileum.

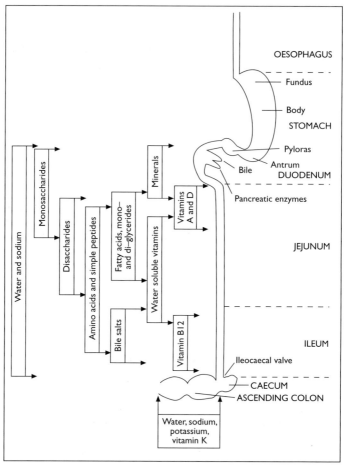

Fig 12.1 Principal absorption sites for nutrients.
With kind permission of Blackwell Science

Transit time in the small intestine is about four to five hours. Foods with a high soluble fibre content, such as oats, pulses, fruit and vegetables, increase transit time, while insoluble fibre found, for example, in wholemeal bread tends to decrease transit time. Natural bran is an insoluble fibre but can reduce the absorption of iron, calcium and zinc.

The indigestible matter then passes into the large intestine. This is approximately one metre long and six centimetres in diameter (MAFF, 1995). Its main function is to absorb water and minerals. A diet high in both soluble and insoluble fibre reduces transit time and gives bulk to the stools, making them easier to pass.

'THE BALANCE OF GOOD HEALTH'

A balanced diet is needed to maintain health, prevent deficiency diseases, keep the immune system functioning efficiently and provide us with energy. It has also been shown to help reduce the risk of developing certain chronic diseases, such as coronary heart disease. 'The Balance of Good Health' is a model to help people make healthy food choices. Foods are divided into five groups relating to their main nutrients. The plate shows the proportions of each food group required to give a balanced diet.

Bread, other cereals and potatoes

This group includes all types of breakfast cereals, bread, pasta, rice, maize, noodles and cornmeal. The main nutrients are complex carbohydrates and B vitamins necessary for energy metabolism. Carbohydrates are broken down to provide energy in the ultimate form of glucose, which is used by all cells in the body and is the sole energy source for the brain.

These starchy foods should constitute the main part of a meal and be eaten at regular intervals during the day. They contain no fat and care should be taken not to increase their fat content, for example, by spreading bread or toast thinly with a low fat spread, using semi-skimmed milk on cereal, and not frying potatoes or adding rich sauces to pasta. Choosing wholemeal or wholegrain varieties provides more fibre which can aid satiety and help prevent constipation.

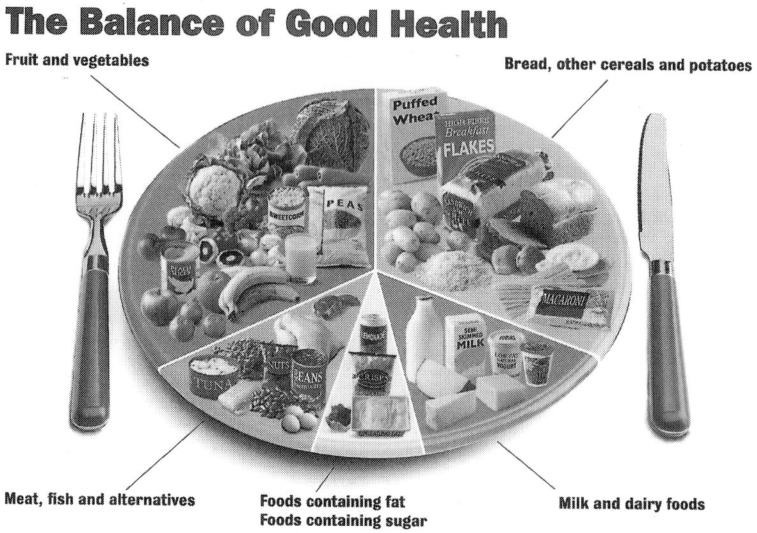

The Balance of Good Health

Fruit and vegetables   Bread, other cereals and potatoes

Meat, fish and alternatives   Foods containing fat   Milk and dairy foods
Foods containing sugar

Fig 12.2 'The Balance of Good Health'.
With kind permission of the Health Education Authority

Fruit and vegetables

This group contains fresh, frozen and tinned fruit and vegetables, dried fruit and fruit juice. The main nutrients provided are vitamin C, fibre, carotenes, folates and many minerals. It is recommended that five portions of fruit and vegetables are eaten daily and that there should be as much variety as possible.

The fibre content of fruit and vegetables varies with the species, part of the plant and its maturity. Fruit and vegetables help to prevent constipation and make excellent snack foods. There is evidence that a high intake of fruit and vegetables is linked with a reduction in the incidence of some cancers and heart disease.

Meat, fish and alternatives

All types of fresh, frozen or tinned meat and fish, poultry, eggs, nuts, beans and pulses are included in this group. Processed foods such as sausages, salami, beefburgers and fish fingers are also included. These provide protein necessary for the growth and renewal of cells, iron, and B vitamins, especially B12, zinc and magnesium. Iron is particularly well absorbed from red meats.

It is preferable to choose lean meat, cut off any fat, remove the skin from poultry and cook without using oil. Beans and pulses are naturally low in fat and provide a useful alternative to meat. It is recommended that no more than two portions are eaten daily. Oily fish, such as mackerel, sardines, salmon, trout and kippers, contain a type of oil that can reduce the viscosity of blood making it less sticky and less likely to clog up the arteries.

Milk and dairy products

This group contains milk, cheese and yoghurt. The main nutrients are calcium, protein, vitamin B12 and vitamins A and D. It is recommended that around one pint of milk is consumed every day, or its equivalent in yoghurt or cheese, where one-third of a pint of milk is equivalent to a small pot of yoghurt or one ounce of hard cheese. This is particularly important for teenagers laying down bone mass and women after the menopause who begin to lose calcium from the bones and run the risk of osteoporosis and bone fractures.

It is wise to choose low fat versions of all dairy products, for example semi-skimmed milk, low fat yoghurt, and cheeses with a lower fat content, such as cottage cheese.

Fatty and sugary foods

This group contains sugar, sweets, chocolate, fizzy drinks, biscuits, cakes, crisps, spreading fats, cooking oils, mayonnaise, rich sauces and more. These foods contain a lot of fat and sugar but relatively few vitamins and minerals. All foods in this group should only be eaten occasionally.

More about fats

The average fat consumption in Great Britain is 42% of total calorie intake. For health reasons it is recommended that total fat intake whatever the type is cut to 35% of total calorie intake (Department of Health, 1991). There are three different types of fat, each with a different effect:

▶ *Saturated fats* found in butter, milk, meat, suet, lard and coconut are generally hard at room temperature and linked with raised cholesterol levels associated with the development of heart disease. It is also thought that trans fats found in many manufactured products, such as cakes, biscuits and some spreading fats have a similar effect.

▶ *Monounsaturated fats* found in olive oil, rapeseed oil and avocado are oils at room temperature and have no effect on cholesterol levels. The amount consumed should not be increased, but it is healthier to swap some saturated fat to monounsaturated fat.

▶ *Polyunsaturated fats* found in sunflower and safflower oil are also oils at room temperature and have been found to lower cholesterol levels, particularly the low density lipoproteins (LDLs) associated with increased risk of heart disease.

Alcohol

It is good to know that this can be included as part of a healthy diet. Studies have shown that taking one to two units of alcohol regularly is beneficial for the heart for men over the age of 40 and women after the menopause. But regular consumption above the recommended level becomes detrimental to health and is linked with raised blood pressure, stroke and liver disease.

The recommended amount for women is two to three units per day and for men is three to four units per day. One day per week should be alcohol free and units should not be saved up for one 'big night'! One unit of alcohol is equal to one pub measure of spirits or half a pint of normal strength lager, cider or beer or one small glass of wine.

Fibre

Fibre is alternatively known as Non Starch Polysaccharide (NSP) (Department of Health, 1991). It is the undigested plant material that ultimately passes into the large intestine. Fibre can be soluble or insoluble; it gives prolonged satiety after a meal and adds bulk to the stools. Insoluble fibre found in wholemeal products has a greater water holding capacity than soluble fibre and it decreases transit time throughout the gut. By contrast, soluble fibre found in fruit, vegetables, beans and oats slows transit in the small intestine, lowers cholesterol levels and slows the absorption of glucose from the gut, so it is particularly beneficial for diabetics and those with raised lipid levels.

THE OSTOMIES

When an ostomy is created, there is loss of continence that can lead to embarrassing social problems, so certain foods may be avoided. Everybody's digestive system reacts differently to different foods and many sources suggest that all foods should be tried on a number of occasions and none specifically avoided.

The colostomy

Colostomy output may be fairly liquid when the colostomy is near to the terminal ileum and more formed when it is nearer to the rectum. A colostomy in the transverse colon produces an output that is paste-like or semi-formed while a left sided or descending colostomy produces a semi-formed or formed output. An end or sigmoid colostomy produces a formed stool because water absorption in the colon is nearly complete.

The colostomate can generally expect timing of motions to be similar to that prior to having a colostomy, with the first motion being initiated by the first meal of the day. Eating regularly will help to predict the timing and number of motions.

Output too liquid

Foods causing loose stools prior to having a colostomy will continue to cause this effect. Some of the foods that most often result in a more liquid output are listed in Table 12.1. Other causes of loose output may be an infection, sorbitol in some sweets or medications, too much dietary fibre or temporary lactose intolerance. Some suggestions to thicken output are given in Table 12.2. If marshmallows are eaten, about twenty are needed to thicken output and individuals should be made aware of the effect this could have on their weight and teeth (Farbrother, 1993).

Table 12.1 Foods that tend to increase output or make output more liquid for colostomates and ileostomates

Diarrhoea/more liquid output	Colostomy	Ileostomy
Alcohol (excess)		Yes
Cabbage	Yes	Yes
Chocolate		Yes
Fish		Yes
Fruit (not banana)	Yes	Yes
Green vegetables	Yes	Yes
Legumes	Yes	Yes
Lettuce		Yes
Nuts		Yes
Oily food		Yes
Onions		Yes
Prunes or prune juice	Yes	Yes
Spicy food	Yes	Yes

Table 12.2 Food that may help to thicken output for colostomates and ileostomates

Thicken output	Colostomy	Ileostomy
Apple sauce	Yes	Yes
Bananas (ripe)	Yes	Yes
Cheese	Yes	Yes
Marshmallows	Yes	Yes
Milk (boiled)	Yes	
Noodles	Yes	
Peanut butter (smooth)	Yes	Yes
Rice (boiled)	Yes	Yes
Tapioca	Yes	Yes

Wind

Gas production varies between one and three litres per day, most of this being ingested! The remainder depends in part on the composition of fibre eaten and the bacterial flora present in the gut.

Every individual has their very own combination of over 400 species of colonic bacteria. Any undigested starch reaching the colon becomes a substrate for these bacteria and they ferment it to produce short chain fatty acids and gas. The main gases produced are carbon dioxide and hydrogen.

Some people also produce methane and hydrogen sulphide. The gut wall can absorb some of these gases which are taken via the bloodstream to the lungs and exhaled. The remaining gas is passed out of the colostomy. It is likely that someone who suffered with wind prior to having a colostomy will continue to have this problem.

Table 12.3 Non food causes of excess wind for all ostomates

Non food causes of wind

1.	Chewing gum
2.	Eating with mouth open
3.	Sucking through a straw
4.	Talking when eating
5.	Smoking
6.	Eating quickly
7.	Eating irregularly or missing meals
8.	Drinking fizzy drinks

There are several non food causes of wind listed in Table 12.3 and these should be checked before blaming a particular food. The foods most often quoted as being gas producers are listed in Table 12.4 and some suggestions to reduce wind in Table 12.5.

Table 12.4 Food items most often associated with excess gas formation for colostomates and ileostomates

Wind	Colostomy	Ileostomy
Beer		Yes
Brussels sprouts	Yes	Yes
Cabbage	Yes	Yes*
Cauliflower	Yes	Yes
Cucumber		Yes
Eggs	Yes	Yes
Green vegetables	Yes*	Yes*
Legumes	Yes*	Yes*
Onions	Yes*	Yes*
Spicy food	Yes	Yes

* Foods most often quoted as wind producers.

Table 12.5 Food items that may help to reduce wind in colostomates and ileostomates

Decreases wind	Colostomy	Ileostomy
Buttermilk	Yes	Yes
Fennel tea	Yes	
Natural yoghurt	Yes	Yes
Peppermint tea	Yes	

It is mainly the fruit and vegetable group that is likely to cause excess gas due to the varying amounts of fibre (NSP) which result in undigested carbohydrates reaching the colon. However, there is no direct linear relation between fibre and gas production (Kramer, 1987). For many health reasons this is the very group that should be increased in the diet. So these foods should be tested at intervals, on several occasions and in different quantities to assess their impact on output.

Odour

Stools have an odour that may vary from day to day. Changing a colostomy bag obviously brings the nose closer to faecal matter than passing faeces per rectum. Some of the foods implicated in producing a strong odour are given in Table 12.6 and suggestions of foods that can help to reduce odour are given in Table 12.7.

Table 12.6 Foods that tend to cause a strong odour in ostomy output

Odour	Colostomy	Ileostomy	Urostomy
Asparagus	Yes		Yes*
Baked beans	Yes	Yes	
Broccoli	Yes	Yes	
Cabbage	Yes		
Cauliflower	Yes		
Cheese		Yes	
Cucumber		Yes	
Eggs		Yes*	
Fish boiled, fried or grilled.	Yes	Yes*	Yes*
Green vegetables	Yes*		
Legumes	Yes		
Onions	Yes	Yes*	

* Foods most often quoted as causing odour in ostomy output.

Table 12.7 Foods that may help to reduce odour in ostomy output

Helps reduce odour	Colostomy	Ileostomy
Buttermilk	Yes	Yes
Yoghurt	Yes	Yes
Peppermint oil		Yes

Constipation

This could cause severe discomfort, poor appetite and stop the colostomy from functioning. Constipation may be a result of immobility, a low fibre diet or some medications. There are three steps to help prevent this occurring:

▶ Increase intake of fruit, vegetables and wholemeal or wholegrain products.

▶ Drink at least eight cups of fluid per day.

▶ Take some gentle exercise daily.

The ileostomy and ileo-anal pouch

The output from an ileostomy is naturally fairly liquid due to the large volume of secretions added to the gut for digestion and the fact that water absorption is incomplete. After ileostomy placement it can take around six weeks or more for the ileum to adapt to absorbing more water. Initial output may be as much as 1500ml per day but over the weeks this reduces to around 600ml–800ml and may have a consistency more like toothpaste. Ileostomates find that their bag usually fills three to four hours after a meal, so to avoid night emptying food intake is usually greater in the morning and tailed off in the afternoon and evening.

It has been reported that ileostomates have a lower dietary intake of fibre, iron and vitamins A and C than a comparable group without an ileostomy (Bingham, 1982). Vitamin B12 deficiency is rare but there is an increased incidence of urinary and bladder stones in ileostomates (McNeil, 1982).

Increased output/diarrhoea

An infection, sorbitol, lactose intolerance or excess fibre may increase output and some of the foods in Table 12.1 may be implicated. Foods that thicken output are listed in Table 12.2. Some foods may be evident, unchanged in the output. This does not mean that the nutrients have not been absorbed, but next time the food is eaten it should be chewed more thoroughly and for longer.

Ileostomy diarrhoea is the term used when output is greater than one litre per day. It may be acute or chronic and dehydration can occur rapidly. Fluid and electrolyte replacement is a priority so salt should be added to food to replace losses in the output. Fluid is better absorbed in the presence of salt so drinks such as Bovril or Marmite are appropriate. An alternative is eating crisps or other salty snacks together with a drink. Isotonic sports drinks are a good option for rehydration, as are rehydration solutions sold over the counter at pharmacies. Alternatively, a rehydration solution can be made at home:

▶ Dissolve half a teaspoon of salt and four teaspoons of sugar in 150ml of water.

▶ Add 150ml of orange juice.

▶ Make this up to 500ml with tap water.

(Garrow and James, 1993)

Wind

Non food causes of wind are the same for ileostomates as colostomates (see Table 12.3). Additionally, bacteria can colonise a small section of the terminal ileum resulting in gas production in the same way as the colon (see Table 12.4).

Blockage

Some foods can temporarily block the narrow ileum causing severe abdominal pain and a non functioning ileostomy. These foods are listed in Table 12.8. The likelihood of blockage is greater if these foods are taken on an empty stomach, for example peanuts before a meal. The blockage is usually related to the amount eaten (Wood, 1998). Until the blockage is dislodged, solid food should be withheld and copious amounts of fluid taken. The offending food should be retested at a later date, perhaps in a smaller quantity, not on its own, ensuring that it is chewed well and not eaten in a hurry.

Table 12.8 Foods that may block an ileostomy, particularly if eaten in large quantities on an empty stomach

Blockage
Celery
Coconut
Dried fruit
Mushrooms
Nuts
Oriental vegetables
Potato skins
Raw fruit skins, pith, pips and stones
Rhubarb
Sweetcorn
Tomato skins

Odour

Certain foods seem to cause odour problems for some people and these are listed in Table 12.6. Ways of reducing odour are shown in Table 12.7.

The ileo-anal pouch

The ileo-anal pouch gives some control over evacuation as the operation creates a pouch for the temporary storage of output. Evacuation will be more frequent than previous bowel motions but can usually be deferred for 20–30 minutes and patients are mainly continent. All the above sections on increased output, diarrhoea, wind, odour and blockage apply to the pouch. In addition, there may be some anal irritants. These are listed in Table 12.9.

Table 12.9 Foods that may cause anal irritation for individuals with an ileo-anal pouch

Anal irritation
Bran
Citrus fruit
Coconut
Oriental vegetables
Popcorn
Spicy food
Sweetcorn

The urostomy/ileal conduit

The urinary system is completely separate from the digestive system. In the kidneys waste products are filtered from the blood forming urine that then passes down the ureters to the urostomy. A high fluid intake will produce more urine and this helps to prevent urinary tract infections.

A healthy fluid intake is between one and a half and two litres per day and this is even more important for the urostomate to help prevent urinary tract infections. The Urostomy Association recommends the consumption of three litres of fluid per day. Intake should be increased in hot weather or if there is more sweating for any reason, for example because of exercise or fever.

Tea, coffee and alcohol are diuretics so drinking these late at night is not a good idea if a good night's sleep is desired. A high vitamin C intake will help to prevent urinary infections by making the urine more acidic. Sources of vitamin C are citrus fruits, such as oranges, grapefruit, mandarins and lemons, soft berries such as blackcurrants, redcurrants and cranberries and squashes like blackcurrant cordial. Research has shown that cranberry juice has particular properties to reduce the incidence of urinary infections and that it only takes one glass per day to confer these benefits.

Odour

This can be a problem for some urostomates and there seem to be two main culprits (see Table 12.6).

Colour

Some foods can give a surprisingly strong colour to the urine, such as those in Table 12.10.

Table 12.10 Foods that may colour output

Colour	Colostomy	Ileostomy	Urostomy
Beetroot	Yes		Yes
Food dyes			Yes
Radishes			Yes
Spinach	Yes	Yes	Yes

Overall a healthy way of eating with all its benefits is achievable by everyone with an ostomy. Some foods may cause certain problems but there is no medical reason that these foods should not be eaten, and nutritionally the more variety in the diet, the greater the chance of achieving a good all round nutritional balance. Many of the problem foods come from the fruit and vegetable group but this group confers many health benefits. So if a certain food seems to be particularly troublesome it should be tried again in a smaller quantity ensuring that it is chewed more thoroughly. A food should not be excluded until it has been retested several times. The food may be tolerated in a smaller quantity or it could be restricted to times when the effect is less embarrassing.

And finally, here are some general tips for people with a stoma:

▶ Enjoy your food, relax when eating and take your time.

▶ Chew food thoroughly.

▶ Eat a wide variety of foods from each of the four main food groups.

▶ Eat at regular times each day to avoid fluctuations in bowel habits.

▶ Avoid under or overeating.

▶ Drink at least eight cups of fluid per day.

▶ Although many fruit and vegetables may cause problems, try to get a good variety.

REFERENCES

Bingham, S. et al (1982) Diet and health of people with an ileostomy: 1. Dietary assessment. *British Journal of Nutrition;* 47: 3, 399–406.

Department of Health (1991) *Dietary Reference Values for Food, Energy and Nutrients.* London: HMSO.

Farbrother, M. (1993) What Can I Eat? *Nursing Times;* 89: 14, 63.

Garrow, J.S., James, W.P.T. (1993) *Human Nutrition and Dietetics.* London: Churchill Livingstone.

Kramer, P. (1987) Effect of specific food, beverages and spices on amount of ileostomy output in human subjects. *The American Journal of Gastroenterology;* 82: 4, 327–332.

MAFF (1995) *Manual of Nutrition.* 10th Edition. London: HMSO.

McNeil, N.I., Bingham, S., Cole, T.J. et al (1982) Diet and health of people with an ileostomy: 2. Ileostomy function and nutritional state. *British Journal of Nutrition;* 47: 3, 407–415.

Wood, S. (1998) Nutrition and Stoma Patients. *Nursing Times;* 94, 65–67.

FURTHER READING

Barker, H.M. (1991) *Beck's Nutrition and Dietetics for Nurses.* 8th Edition. London: Churchill Livingstone.

Groff, J.L., Groppel, S.S., Hunt, S.M. et al (1995) *Advanced Nutrition and Human Metabolism.* St Paul, USA: West Publishing Co.

Health Education Authority (1994) *The Balance of Good Health.* London: HEA Publishing.

Thomas, B. (1994) *Manual of Dietetic Practice.* Oxford: Blackwell Science Ltd.

Vander, A.J., Sherman, J.H., Luciano, D.S. (1994) *Human Physiology.* New York, NY: McGraw Hill Inc.

Wade, B. (1989) *A Stoma is for Life.* London: Scutari Press.

Appendix A

Drugs and the effect on stomas

Nicholas M. Carter

Administration of drugs requires a little more thought with ostomy patients compared with the average patient. The majority of drugs are absorbed into the blood stream via the stomach, which will obviously not be altered in the ostomy patient. However many drugs are now designed to have a modified release system in order to improve patient compliance. These groups of drugs need a little more thought before prescribing to ostomists.

The first group of modified release drugs to look at is the enteric–coated drugs, for example prednisolone e/c 5mg tablets. These drugs have a special coating applied to them, which allows the tablet to pass unaffected through the stomach, having an acid medium and then, in the less acidic medium of the lower parts of the gastrointestinal tract, the coating allows dissolution of the tablet and release of the drug. This method of drug release will be affected in the ostomy patient to the point where they are not suitable for them. If the drug is formulated like this in order to protect the stomach, an alternative drug may be required. If this style of drugs were to be used, they would be excreted via the stoma without being absorbed by the body.

The second group of drugs to consider is the slow release capsules, for example Slo-phyllin 250mg capsules. These are tiny pellets of drugs with coatings of varying thickness. The coatings take a longer time to dissolve depending on their thickness, so the body has a steady stream of drug available to it over a period of time. These pellets are held together in a gelatin capsule, not suitable for the ostomy patient, and again tend to pass straight out of the body via the stoma.

The third group of drugs is known as modified release drugs and these are indicated as 's/r' or 'm/r' in their description. This type of formulation is becoming more widely used to reduce the frequency of dosage for the patient, hence improving their compliance, for example isosorbide mononitrate 60mg s/r tablets. This style of formulation is often applied to drugs involved in reducing high blood pressure so compliance is important. The drug is formulated within a waxy matrix, the effect being that the drug takes a long time to release and the tablet passes a long way through the gastrointestinal tract. This formulation will not be suitable since, again, it will be excreted via the stoma largely untouched. Some of this group have a slightly different formulation in that the tablets are pressed out with a higher compression ratio. This gives a 'hard' tablet which dissolves only slightly slower than a normal release tablet, for example nifedipine 20mg m/r tablets. These tablets may be suitable for some ostomy patients.

Drugs that do not have modified release formulations can also require a little more consideration before prescribing to ostomy patients. The shortened gastrointestinal tract can alter a drug's therapeutic effect. Some drugs act by reabsorption from the colon – in the ostomy patient this will not happen. Oral contraceptive drugs operate via this mechanism so are not suitable for most ostomy patients. Diuretic drugs can be used with caution. The drugs work by forcing the kidneys to excrete more water. In the normal gastrointestinal tract the actual fluid loss is compensated for by reabsorption from the colon in large amounts. This will not be so in the ostomy patient so the effect of the diuretic will be greatly enhanced for these patients and dehydration will occur more rapidly.

Some of the prescribed drugs may have an effect on the output from the stoma. Certain drugs can reduce the output by slowing down the muscles, for example loperamide; others can increase the output leading to diarrhoea, for example ampicillin; and some will change the colour of the output, which may lead to patient concern, for example indomethacin.

DRUGS INCREASING OUTPUT FROM THE STOMA

Antibiotics

These drugs kill off bacteria within the gut thereby altering the balance that normally exists. This allows increased growth of the remaining bacteria and can lead to a diarrhoea attack. Examples include amoxycillin, ampicillin, flucloxacillin, erythromycin and penicillin. There are no antibiotics available for sale over the counter in the UK, but they may be purchased in some other countries where restrictions are different.

Magnesium containing antacids

The magnesium parts of these drugs have an osmotic effect in the gastrointestinal tract that increases the water content of stools and leads to diarrhoea, for example magnesium trisilicate mixture. If a combined magnesium and aluminium based product, such as Mucogel or Maalox, is chosen the problem can be overcome.

Iron preparations

The iron preparations will lead to loose motions through the stoma. Examples are ferrous sulphate, ferrous gluconate, Feospan, Fefol, Pregaday, Ferrograd, Fersamal and many multivitamin and mineral preparations.

Sugar free products

The sweeteners used in many sugar free products can have an osmotic effect on the gut as described under 'magnesium containing antacids' above. This leads to a more fluid output from the stoma. The sweeteners to be aware of are mannitol and sorbitol.

Metoclopramide and domperidone

These two drugs are used to reduce nausea in patients, the metoclopramide being available only on prescription either as a generic or as Maxolon. Domperidone is available as Motilium both on and off prescription. They work by increasing gastric motility and speeding up the movement of the stomach contents through the gut. This may lead to increased output from the stoma.

Proton pump inhibitors

The drugs in this group are only given on prescription and the side effect that concerns the ostomy patient is the production of diarrhoea. The drugs are omeprazole, Losec, lansoprazole, Zoton, pantoprazole, Protium and, the newest one, Pariet.

Drugs reducing output from the stoma

Analgesics

Ordinary, simple pain killers such as paracetamol, aspirin or ibuprofen will have no effect on output from the stoma. However many 'stronger' preparations use these basic ingredients combined with opioid derivatives, for example co-codamol containing paracetamol and codeine. The opioid is added to enhance the analgesic effect of the paracetamol, aspirin or ibuprofen. The side effect of the opioid that concerns the ostomy patient is the reduction in gut motility creating a constipating effect, thus reducing output. The drugs falling in this category are codeine, morphine, dextropropoxyphene and dihydrocodeine. They are used in a variety of combinations and strengths in a large number of drugs both on prescription and over the counter.

▶ Co-codamol – paracetamol and codeine in a variety of strengths, available as Paracodol, Kapake, Solpadol and Tylex on prescription and as Paracodol, Panadeine, Solpadeine, Veganin, Syndol, Solpadeine Max, Panadol Ultra and Migraleve for sale through pharmacies. (There are many others not listed here.)

▶ Co-dydramol – paracetamol and dihydrocodeine in a variety of strengths available as Remedeine and Remedeine forte on prescription and as Paramol over the counter.

▶ Co-proxamol – paracetamol and dextropropoxyphene, also referred to as 'Distalgesic' by patients. This combination is not available for sale.

As well as the above combinations with paracetamol as the basic drug, there are other combinations of aspirin and ibuprofen with an opioid derivative, again to enhance the pain killing effect.

▶ Co-codaprin – aspirin and codeine in combination available as a generic formulation as solid or soluble tablets. Also available over the counter as Veganin or Codis.

▶ Ibuprofen and codeine – this has no 'approved name' but is becoming much more widely available over the counter. The recent regulations restricting sizes of paracetamol and aspirin products that can be sold to the public do not apply to ibuprofen based products. This means that the manufacturers can sell large sizes of products in this group making it a more lucrative market. On prescription the product is available as Codafen Continus, a slow release product containing 20mg codeine. Over the counter the products currently available are Nurofen Plus and Solpaflex.

This is probably the largest area of drugs that can reduce stoma output and care must be taken when prescribing for prescription or over the counter.

Bulk forming laxatives

The bulk forming laxatives are fibre laxatives that reduce stoma output by increasing the volume of the stools. In liquid form there is lactulose, known either generically or by its trade names, which include Duphalac, Lactugal, and Regulose. It is available as a pre-packed over the counter product. There is also a sachet form available, prescribed as lactulose dry or Duphalac Dry. More commonly used to slow down the stoma action are the fibre products such as Fybogel, Isogel, Regulan, Movicol, Normacol and Manevac, although the latter also contains some senna. These products taken with a smaller amount of water than recommended in the instructions will lead to a reduction in stoma output which at times may be of some use.

Antimotility drugs

These drugs are used to reduce diarrhoea in the non-ostomy patient. They act directly on the smooth muscle in the bowel reducing movement and allowing stool formation to occur. The introduction of these drugs to the ostomy patient could have a much-enhanced effect, reducing stoma output severely. This group contains:

- Codeine, which has a constipating action when given in higher doses on its own. This is available as a generic, or as Diarrest on prescription.
- Co-phenotrope, a combination of diphenoxylate and atropine available only on prescription as Lomotil.
- Loperamide, available as generic both on and off prescription in capsule, syrup and tablet form. It is available under a wide variety of over the counter names including Arret, Diasorb, Diocalm Ultra, Diahlimit, Imodium and Imodium Plus.
- Morphine, available as 'kaolin and morphine', J Collis Browne's Mixture and Tablets, Enterosan and Diocalm.

Antimuscarinic drugs

These are sometimes less correctly called anticholinergic drugs. They are used to reduce gut motility, which is sometimes required in a patient. They reduce the contractions within the smooth muscle in the lower gastrointestinal tract, slowing down stoma output. Again these drugs are available on prescription and over the counter in different products. Examples include dicyclomine, available as Merbentyl on prescription, although it is also possible to purchase it from pharmacies as Kolanticon Gel. Hyoscine is available both on and off prescription as Buscopan tablets.

Antispasmodic drugs

This group has always been available on prescription and now has also had been switched to a P. licence enabling pharmacy led sales. Drugs in this group have been heavily advertised on television and patients may not be aware of what they are buying. They relax the smooth muscle in the bowel in order to reduce the pain and bloating effect caused by 'Irritable Bowel Syndrome'. This mode of action will reduce stoma output.

- Alverine citrate, known as Spasmonal on prescription and also available as Relaxyl for over the counter sales.
- Mebeverine hydrochloride, on prescription as generic or as Colofac and also available over the counter as Equilon or Colofac.
- Peppermint oil capsules, Colpermin or Mintec available both on and off prescription and Equilon Herbal purely for sale.

Tricyclic antidepressant drugs

These drugs can have a constipating effect on the bowel thus reducing stoma output. This side effect is caused by the antimuscarinic activity of these drugs (see above for more details). Only available on prescription, these drugs include amitriptyline, Tryptizol, Triptafen, clomipramine, Anafranil, dothiepin, Prothiaden, imipramine, lofepramine, Gamanil and mianserin.

Antimuscarinic drugs and parkinsonism

Antimuscarinic drugs are used in treatment of the tremor symptoms of parkinsonism. The side effects of these are as mentioned earlier so if these drugs are used the prescriber must be aware of the patient's needs. The main drugs used in this manner are benzhexol, Artane, benztropine, Cogentin, orphenadrine and procyclidine.

H2-receptor antagonists

These drugs are available for sale and on prescription. They do have side effects that alter bowel habit but there is no clear alteration one way or the other. In some patients they can produce diarrhoea yet in others they cause constipation. I have made reference to them since they are now widely available over the counter. Products include cimetidine, Tagamet, famotidine, Pepcid, ranitidine, Zantac, nizatidine and Axid.

Antihistamines

The main drug to consider here is chlorpheniramine, or Piriton, one of the older style antihistamines causing sedation. It has antimuscarinic side effects reducing output from the stoma.

Beta-blockers

One of the side effects of these drugs can be constipation leading to reduced stoma output. This group includes propranolol, Inderal, atenolol, Tenormin, bisoprolol, Monocor, Emcor, carvedilol, Eucardic, celiprolol, Celectol, metoprolol and Betaloc.

COLOUR CHANGES IN STOMA OUTPUT DUE TO DRUGS

Strictly speaking these drugs will cause colour changes in faeces and urine in both ostomy and non ostomy patients, but due to their awareness of stoma output it may be a little more worrying for the ostomy patient.

- Antacids containing aluminium – these can cause white or grey specks in the faeces.
- Antibiotics – green or grey output.
- Anticoagulants – pink to red to black output.
- Iron salts – black output.
- Indomethacin – green output.
- Senna – yellow-green to brown output.

Drugs causing colour changes in urine

- Amitriptyline – changes urine to blue green colour.
- Iron salts – black urine.
- Ibuprofen – red urine.
- Indomethacin – green urine.
- Methyldopa – darkens urine.
- Metronidazole – red to brown urine.

- Nitrofurantoin – brown to yellow.
- Senna – yellow-brown or pink urine.
- Triamterene – (a diuretic) blue urine.
- Warfarin – orange urine.

There are many potential problems with drugs and their side effects but with a little thought these problems can be overcome or at least explained.

FURTHER READING

British National Formulary, March 1999. B.M.A. Royal Pharmaceutical Society. UK.

Skelton, J. (1999) Chemist and Druggist Guide to O.T.C. (14th edition) UK: Miller Freeman.

Bowman, W.C., Rand, M.J. (1982) Textbook of Pharmacology. (2nd edition) Cambridge: University Press Cambridge.

Alexander, A., Anderson, C. (1991) *The Pharmaceutical Journal*; November 23, 1991, 698-699.

Appendix B
Useful addresses

APPLIANCE
MANUFACTURERS

B.Braun Biotrol S.A.
Parkway Close
Parkway Industrial Estate
Sheffield S9 4WJ
Tel: 0114 270 2391
Fax: 0114 279 6709
Email:
b.braun.biotrol@dial.pipex.com

Coloplast Ltd
Peterborough Business Park
Peterborough PE2 6FX
Tel: 0800 220622
Email: stomacare@coloplast.com
www.coloplast.com

Convatec Ltd
Harrington House
Milton Road
Ickenham
Uxbridge UB10 8PU
Tel: 0800 282254

Dansac Ltd
Victory House
Vision Park
Histon
Cambridge CB4 4ZR
Tel: 01223 235100
Fax: 01223 235146

Hollister Ltd
Rectory Court
42 Broad Street
Wokingham
Berkshire RG40 1GZ
Tel: 0800 521377

Marlen (UK) Ltd
Unit F4C, Keighley Business
Centre
South Street
Keighley BD21 1AG
Tel: 0800 317602
Fax: 01535 611088

Oakmed Ltd
54 Adams Avenue
Northampton NN1 4LJ
Tel: 01604 239250
Fax: 01604 629713

Pelican Healthcare Ltd
Cardiff Business Park
Cardiff CF4 1ZZ
Tel: 0800 318282
Fax: 029 20747001

Salts Healthcare
Lord Street
Birmingham B7 4DS
Tel: 0121 359 5123
Fax: 0121 359 0830

Simms Portex Ltd
Hythe
Kent CT21 6JL
Tel: 0800 525350
Fax: 01303 265560

Welland Medical Ltd
7/8 Brunel Centre
Newton Road
Crawley
West Sussex. RH10 2TU
Tel: 01293 615455
Fax: 01293 615412

Distributed by:
Clinimed Ltd UK
Tel: 01628 850100
Fax: 01628 850331
www.clinimed.co.uk

SUPPORT GROUPS

**Spina Bifida Association for
Spina Bifida and Hydrocephalus
(ASBAH)**
42 Park Road
Peterborough PE1 2UQ
Tel: 01733 555988
Fax: 01733 555985
Email:
postmaster@asbah.demon.co.uk.

British Colostomy Association
15 Station Road
Reading RG1 1LG
Tel: 0118 939 1537
Email: sue@bcass.org.uk

**Ileostomy and Internal Pouch
Association**
PO Box 132
Scunthorpe DN15 9YW
Tel: 01724 720150

**National Association for Colitis
and Crohn's Disease (NACC)**
PO Box 205
St Albans
Herts. AL1 1AB
Tel: 01727 844296
Email: nacc@nacc.org.uk

Red Lion Group
20 The Maltings
Green Lane
Ashwell
Herts. SG7 5LW
*This is a support network for people
with internal pouches*

Spinal Injuries Association
76 St James's Lane
London N10 3DF
Tel: 020 8444 2121

Urostomy Association
Buckland
Beaumont Park
Danbury
Essex CM3 4DE
Tel: 01245 224294

DRUG COMPANIES ALLIED TO STOMA CARE

SmithKline Beecham
Welwyn Garden City
Herts. AL7 1EY
Tel: 01707 325111
Supplies patient information leaflets

Zeneca Pharma
Kings Court
Water Lane
Wilmslow
Cheshire SK9 5AZ
Tel: 01625 712434
Fax: 01625 712530
Provides patient information booklets

CANCER RELATED ADDRESSES

BACUP
3 Bath Place
London EC2A 3JR.
Tel: 020 7696 9003

Cancerlink
11–21 Northdown Street
London N1 9BN
Tel: 020 7833 2818

Cancer Research Campaign
10 Cambridge Terrace
London NW1 4JL
Tel: 020 7224 1333

Colon Cancer Concern
4 Rickett Street
London SW6 1RU
Tel: 020 7381 4711 (Info Line)
Fax: 020 7381 5752

Crocus Trust
Tel: 0870 242 4870
Promotes the symptoms of colorectal cancer

Imperial Cancer Research Fund
PO Box 123
Lincoln's Inn Fields
London WC2A 3PX
Tel: 020 7242 0200

Macmillan Cancer Relief
Anchor House
15–19 Bitten Street
London SW3 3TZ
Tel: 020 7351 7811

Marie Curie Cancer Care
28 Belgrave Square
London SW1X 8OG
Tel: 020 7235 3225

PAEDIATRIC STOMA AND ASSOCIATED SUPPORT GROUPS

National Advisory Service for Parents of Children with a Stoma and associated bowel management problems (NASPCS)
Mr J.B. Malcolm – National Organiser
51 Anderson Drive
Valley View Park
Darvel
Ayrshire KA17 0DE
Tel: 01560 22024

Crohn's in Childhood Research Association
Parkgate House
356 West Barnes Lane
Motspur Park
Surrey KT3 6NB
Tel: 020 8949 6209

Down's Syndrome Association
155 Mitcham Road
London SW17 9PG
Tel: 020 8682 4001
Fax 020 8682 4012

Scottish Down's Syndrome Association
158–160 Balgreen Road
Edinburgh EH11 3AU
Tel: 0131 313 4225
Fax: 0131 313 4285

Down's Heart Group
17 Cantilupe Close
Eaton Bray
Dunstable LU6 2EA
Tel: 01525 220379
Fax: 01525 221553

Gut Motility Disorders Support Network
7 Walden Road
Sewards End
Saffron Walden CB10 2LE
Tel: 01799 520580 (evenings)
Telephone support network

GEEPS – Abdominal Exstrophies (Gastroschisis, Exomphalos or Exstrophies)
104 Riversdale Road,
Romford RM5 2NS
Tel: 01708 738134

**Vater Association and TOFS
(Tracho Oesphageal Fistula
Society)**
St George's Centre
91 Victoria Road
Netherfield
Nottingham NG4 2NN
Tel: 0115 940 0694

**Spina Bifida Association for
Spina Bifida and Hydrocephalus
(ASBAH)**
42 Park Road
Peterborough PE1 2UQ
Tel: 01733 555988
Fax: 01733 555985
Email:
postmaster@asbah.demon.co.uk.

Scottish Spina Bifida Association
190 Queensferry Road
Edinburgh EH4 2BW.
Tel: 0131 332 0743
Fax: 0131 343 3651
Email: ssbahq@compuserve.com

**The Enuresis Resource and
Information Centre (ERIC)**
34 Old School House
Britannia Road
Kingswood
Bristol BS15 2DB
Tel: 0117 960 3060
Fax: 0117 960 0401

Network 81
1–7 Woodfield Terrace
Chapel Hill
Stansted
Essex EM24 8AJ
Tel: 01279 647415
Fax: 01279 816438
*A national network of parents of
children with special educational
needs, offering information guidance,
help and advice on the Education
Acts, other legislation and
administrative practices concerned
with special educational provision*

The Family Fund Trust
PO Box 50
York Y91 9ZS
Tel: 01904 621115
Fax: 01904 658085
*For families with severely disabled
children*

Contact a Family
Contact Line: 020 7383 3555
*A national helpline through which
parent advisers answer telephone or
written inquiries from parents and
professionals on any topic relating to
children's disabilities and the welfare
of the families. Families can be linked
to the appropriate groups or linked on
a one to one basis.*

SOURCES OF HELP AND SUPPORT FOR RELATIONSHIP PROBLEMS

BACUP
3 Bath Place
London EC2A 3JR.
Tel: 020 7696 9003

British Association for Counselling (BAC)
1 Regent Place
Rugby CV21 2PJ
Tel: 01788 578328

British Association of Sexual and Marital Therapy
PO Box 62
Sheffield S10 3TS

British Colostomy Association
15 Station Road
Reading RG1 1LG
Tel: 01734 391537
Email: sue@bcass.org.uk

Carers National Association
Ruth Pitter House
20–25 Glasshouse Yard
London EC1 1LG
Tel: 020 7490 8898 (Mon–Fri 1–4pm)

Compassionate Friends
53 North Street
Bedminster
Bristol B53 1EN
Tel: 0117 966 5202
Helpline: 0117 953 9639

Crossroads Caring for Carers
10 Regents Place
Rugby CV21 2PN
Tel: 01788 573653

Cruse – Bereavement care
Cruse House
126 Sheen Road
Richmond
Surrey TW9 1UR
Tel: 020 8940 4818

Gay Ostomists Association
72 Tramway Road
Liverpool L17 7AZ
Tel: 0151 726 9019

Ileostomy and Internal Pouch Association
PO Box 132
Scunthorpe DN15 9YW
Tel: 01724 720150

Impotence Information Centre
PO Box 1130
London W3 9BB

Institute of Psychosexual Medicine
Lettsom House
11 Chandos Street
London W1M 9DE
Tel: 020 7580 0631

London Lesbian and Gay Switchboard
PO Box 7324
London N1 9QS
Tel: 020 7837 7324

Marie Stopes International
108 Whitfield Street
London W1P 6BE
Tel: 020 7388 0662

Relate
Herbert Gray College
Little Church Street
Rugby CV21 3AP
Tel: 01788 573241

Samaritans
10 The Grove
Slough SL1 1QP
Tel: 0345 909090

SPOD (Sexual problems of the disabled)
286 Camden Street
London N7 0BJ

MISCELLANEOUS ADDRESSES

Age Concern
Astral House
1268 London Road
London SW16 4ER
Tel: 020 8679 8000

British Digestive Foundation
PO Box 251
Edgware HA8 6HG

Help the Aged
St James Walk
Clerkenwell Green
London EC1R 0BE
Tel: 020 7253 0253

Institute of Complementary Medicine
PO Box194
London SE16 1QZ
Tel: 020 7237 5165

The Pain Society
9 Bedford Square
London WC1B 3RA
Tel: 020 7636 2750
Fax: 020 7323 2015
Email: painsoc@compuserve.com

The Patients' Association
PO Box 935
Harrow
Middlesex HA1 3YJ
Tel: 020 8423 8999

Videos for Patients Ltd
68a Delancey Street
London NW1 7RY
Tel: 020 7284 0242
Fax: 020 7284 1004

U.T. Care Products Ltd
The Brampton Centre
Brampton Road
Wath-upon-Dearne
Rotherham S63 6BB
Tel: 01709 872137
Fax: 01709 760073
Suppliers of Valley Cushions.

NURSING

Royal College of Nursing
29 Cavendish Square
London W1M 0BE
Tel: 020 7409 3535

The Queens Nursing Institute
3 Abermarle Way
London EC1V 4JB
Tel: 020 7490 4227

World Council of Enterostomal
Therapists
WCET Central Office
PO Box 48099
60 Dundas Street East
Mississauga
Ontario L5A 4G8
Canada
Tel: +1 905 848 9400
Fax: +1 905 848 9413

This page can be photocopied for your own use

LOCAL ADDRESSES

LOCAL STOMA CARE NURSE

Name:

Address:

Tel:

LOCAL SUPPORT GROUP

Name:

Contact:

LOCAL CHEMIST

Name:

Address:

Tel:

LOCAL APPLIANCE DELIVERY COMPANY

Name:

Address:

Tel:

Stoma Care in the Community. Published by NT Books, 2000.

Index